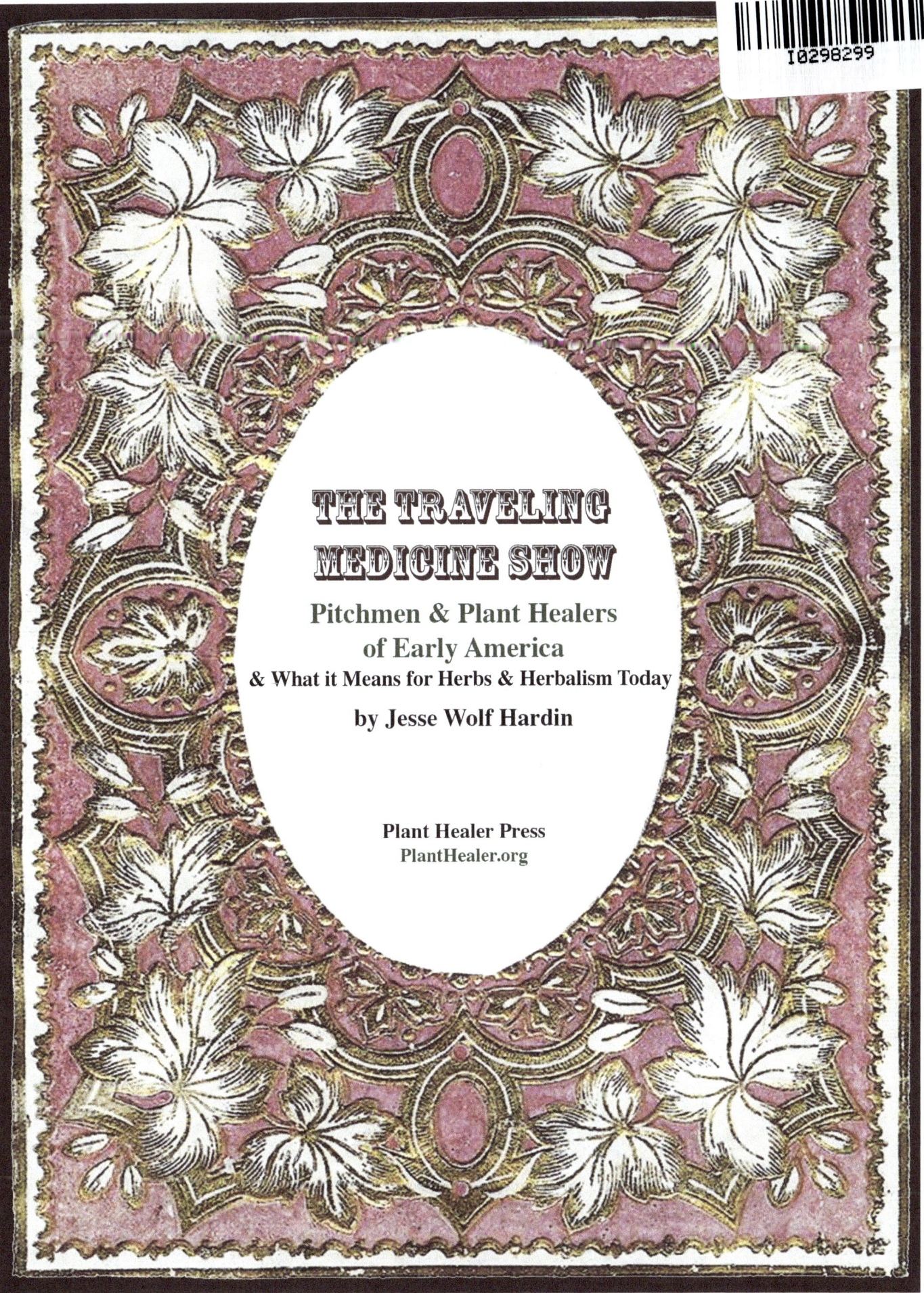

# THE TRAVELING MEDICINE SHOW

## Pitchmen & Plant Healers of Early America
### & What it Means for Herbs & Herbalism Today

by Jesse Wolf Hardin

Plant Healer Press
PlantHealer.org

# THE KICKAPOO DOCTOR

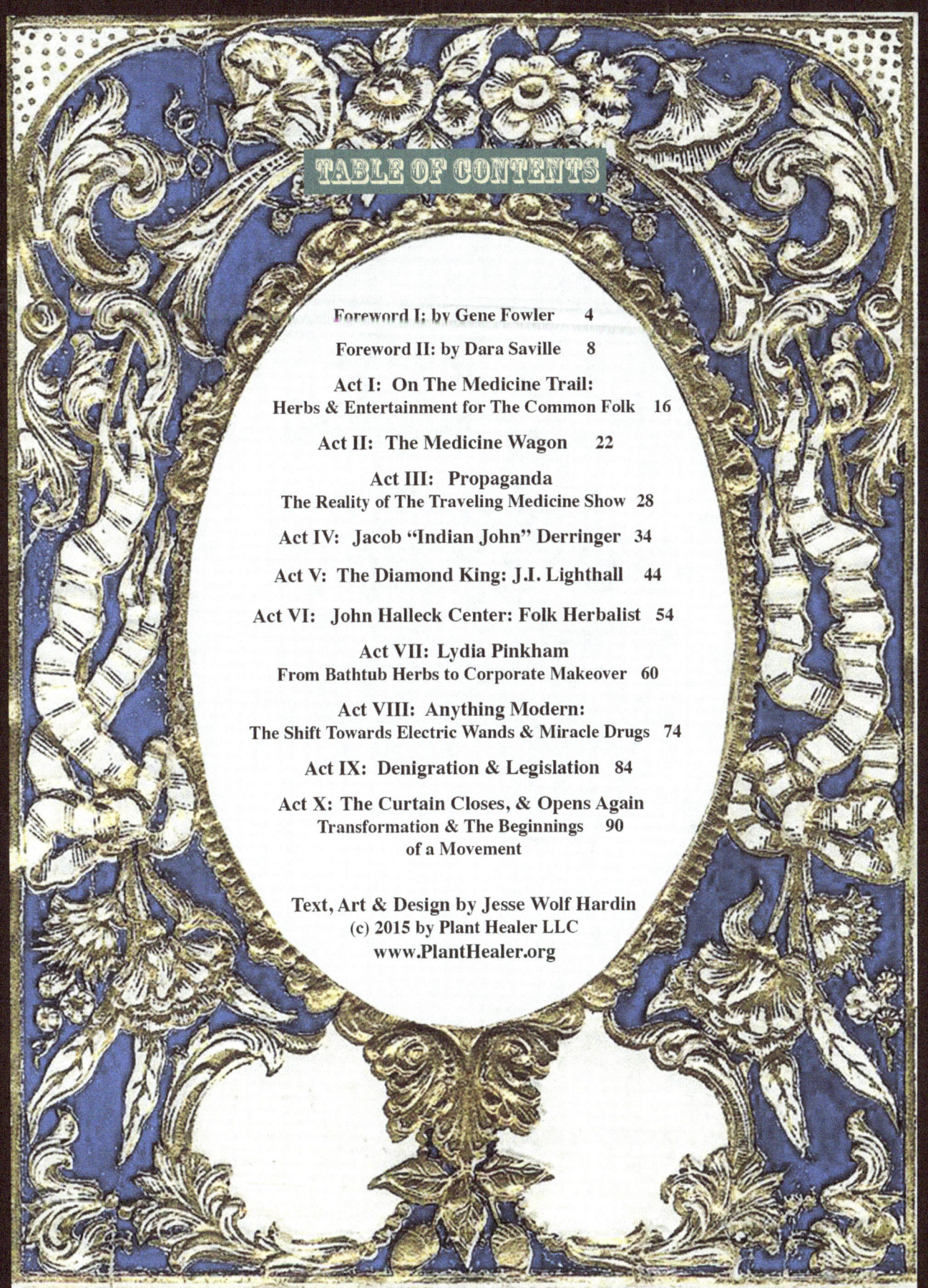

## TABLE OF CONTENTS

Foreword I: by Gene Fowler  4

Foreword II: by Dara Saville  8

**Act I: On The Medicine Trail:**
Herbs & Entertainment for The Common Folk  16

**Act II:** The Medicine Wagon  22

**Act III: Propaganda**
The Reality of The Traveling Medicine Show  28

**Act IV:** Jacob "Indian John" Derringer  34

**Act V:** The Diamond King: J.I. Lighthall  44

**Act VI:** John Halleck Center: Folk Herbalist  54

**Act VII: Lydia Pinkham**
From Bathtub Herbs to Corporate Makeover  60

**Act VIII: Anything Modern:**
The Shift Towards Electric Wands & Miracle Drugs  74

**Act IX:** Denigration & Legislation  84

**Act X: The Curtain Closes, & Opens Again**
Transformation & The Beginnings  90
of a Movement

Text, Art & Design by Jesse Wolf Hardin
(c) 2015 by Plant Healer LLC
www.PlantHealer.org

# FOREWORD

## by Gene Fowler

Obsessions. Most of us have them. They make life peppier and more interesting. But once you have one, it can be hard as heck to figure out where it came from. Among other things, I'm obsessed with the old-time medicine shows, that exotic niche of American showbiz that combined nostrum-selling and mending the mortal chassis with a wide variety of entertainment.

How I got this way I got no clue. But I have learned that, like most things, the medicine shows were not uniformly what they seem in the shorthand of the culture-at-large. The "physic operas" were not always the low-down, dopey scams depicted in story and lore. While the med-show underground certainly harbored its share of con artists, there were also many healing thespians hawking respectable remedies who tried to deliver an experience of wellness and wonder. Even in cases where the medicine sold didn't do all that was promised (as was also sometimes the case with more "mainstream" meds sold in 19th and early 20th century drugstores, some of which contained dangerous levels of morphine, opium, etc.), the show itself delivered a placebo effect, lifting folks' spirits and, consequently, helping the body to heal itself.

Many med-show elixirs, of course, were derived from plants, drawing on herbal traditions of Native America, the Old World, and the mystic distant Orient. The mesmerizing orators who ballyhooed their healing powers were alt-med pioneers. Today even the most austere physician will generally concur that some plant-based medicines are efficacious remedies. And few would deny that there is a connection between the mind, the emotions, and the relative well-being of the earthly vessel in which such mysteries are lodged.

All of which encourages a reconsideration of the American medicine show. In addition to the showfolks' preaching of the gospel of natural healing, I think one of the reasons Jesse Wolf Hardin finds the subject interesting is one of the same reasons that I have spent far more time and energy researching it than would a slightly saner man. The medicine show personalities were colorful, intriguing figures who took advantage of the vast stage for self-invention availing all in the twilight years of the American frontier. They had names like Yellowstone Kit, Diamond Dick, Nevada Ned, Rolling Thunder, Dakota Jack, Oregon Charley, Kansas Charley, Texas Charley, and Dr. Blue Mountain Joe. Their personages were spectacles of hair, hats, buckskin, jewels, and glittering raiment of all manner and description. The medicines they sold bespoke a showiness all their own – Wizard Oil, Kickapoo Worm Killer, Nez Perce Catarrh Snuff, and Warm Springs Consumption Cure. Life on the road with a medicine show could be hard, but it could also be romantic, wild, and free.

I've been researching the life and career of medicine showman extraordinaire J.I. Lighthall, aka the Great Indian Medicine Man of Peoria and aka The Diamond King, whom Hardin includes here, for a quarter of a century. The fact that he died in 1886, just days after his 30th birthday, and the fact that med-show performers flourished in a less-documented quarter of American culture than, say, opera singers, has made tracking the dazzling doc an intriguing challenge. Still, much has been discovered.

His 1882 book, for instance, The Indian Household Medicine Guide, has been reprinted at least a half-dozen times. The title page of the 1882 edition shares authorship with Dr. W.O. Davis, an 1879 graduate of the Eclectic Medical Institute of Cincinnati. (The reissues all reprint the 1883 edition, which deleted Davis' name.) I included some of Lighthall's and Davis' medical formulas in the appendix of my 1997 book, Mystic Healers and Medicine Shows. Based on those excerpts and on my chapter about Lighthall, British pharmacy professor and historian Raymond C. Rowe testified in a 2003 issue of the International Journal of Pharmaceutical Medicine that Lighthall "had a reasonable knowledge of 19th century medicine and materia medica." Analyzing Lighthall's use of Buchu, Uva Ursi, Eucalyptus, Juniper berries, White Oak bark, and other plant components, the professor judged the showman to have been "anything but a charlatan."

After the Diamond King died of smallpox, contracted from the crowd at his performance on Military Plaza in San Antonio, his resourceful widow Victoria, aka "Mrs. Doctor Lighthall," headed up the traveling caravan of medicine-selling entertainers for another decade or so. On an 1889 trek through the Territory of New Mexico, the Las Cruces Daily News advertised that the "celebrated Indian Remedies" ballyhooed by the troupe "are guaranteed strictly vegetable and sold under a guarantee to give satisfaction if used according to directions." Furthermore, Mrs. Dr. Lighthall announced that "$500 will be paid anyone showing that chloroform or opiates of any kind are used in the preparation" of her late husband's medicines.

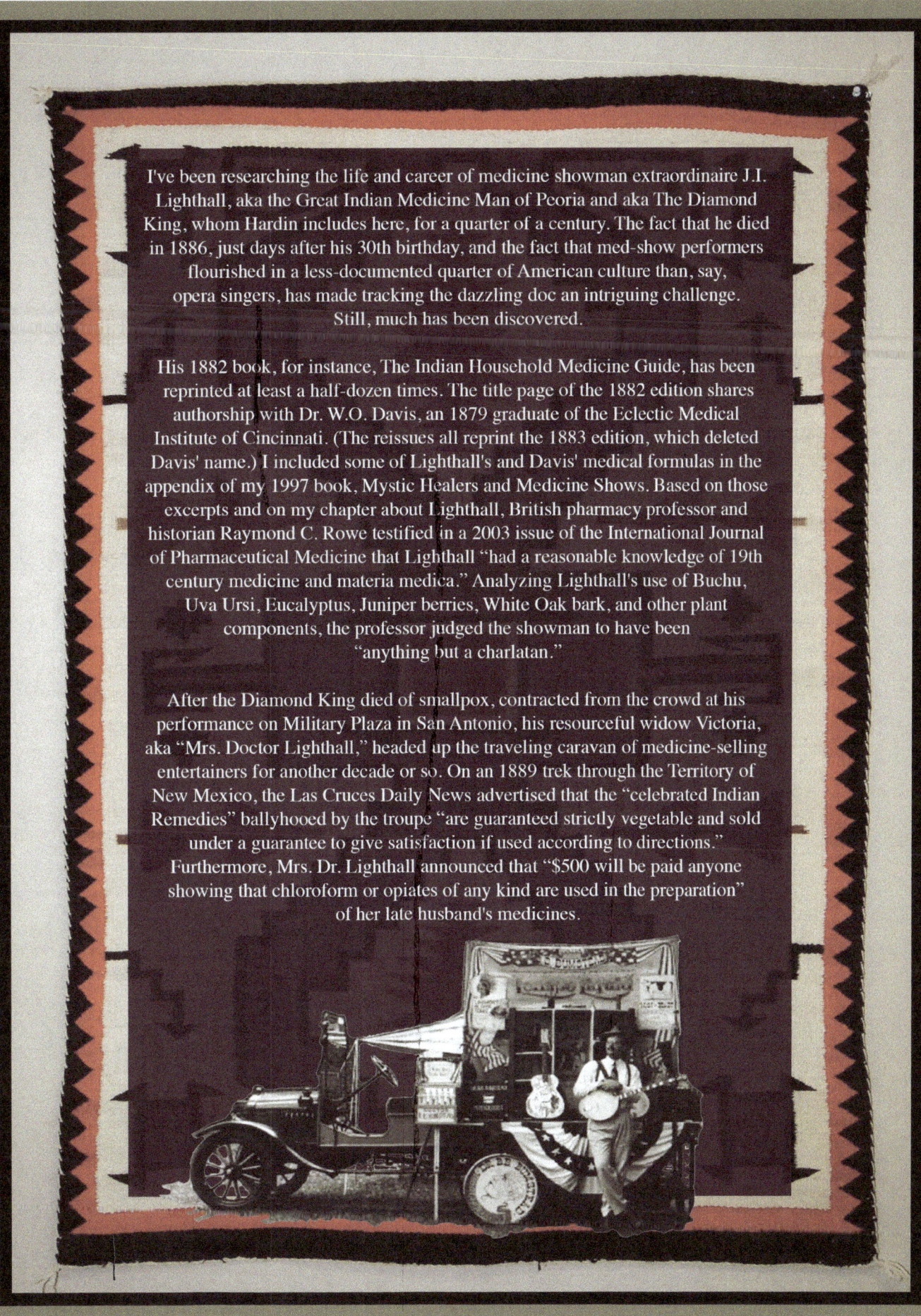

These days—21st century American culture being what it is—in addition to reprints of his book, you can find the Diamond King's image all over the Internet, as e-marketers hawk posters, notecards, key chains, ball caps, and coffee mugs emblazoned with a brightly-colorized cabinet photo of Lighthall, taken in St. Louis in 1885. The medicine man wears an ornate sombrero, an Indian head nickel necklace, and festive duds that seem rustled from the wardrobe of a latter-day alt-country rocker.

I suspect, however, that Doc Lighthall would like to be remembered for his medicines as much as his fashionistahood. As he versified in his household guide:

It's made of barks, and oils, and leaves,
And seldom ever man deceives.
It never fails to satisfy,
And on it, friends, you can rely.

It cures your aches, it cures your pains,
And everywhere an honor gains.
The way it cures it does beat all –
It's made and sold by J. Lighthall.

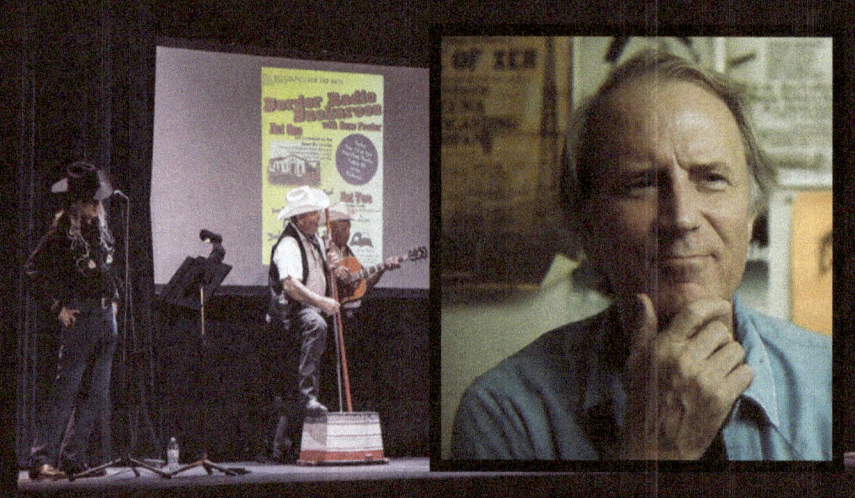

**Gene Fowler** *has written about medicine shows in* True West, Texas Highways, Journal of Texas Music History, *and* Cowboys & Indians. *His books include* Mavericks, Crazy Water, *and* Border Radio. *He is currently working on an extended, semi-fictionalized narrative about the Diamond King, and he is also collaborating on an illustrated history of the American medicine show with Raleigh, North Carolina med-show enthusiast Marshall Wyatt. Wyatt's indie label, Old Hat Records, issued* Good For What Ails You, *a two-CD set of 1920s and '30s med-show music with 70-page booklet. As a performer, Gene Fowler's appearances have included the Kennedy Center, the San Antonio Rodeo, Contemporary Arts Museum Houston, the White Elephant Saloon of Fort Worth, and the Nashville Network.*

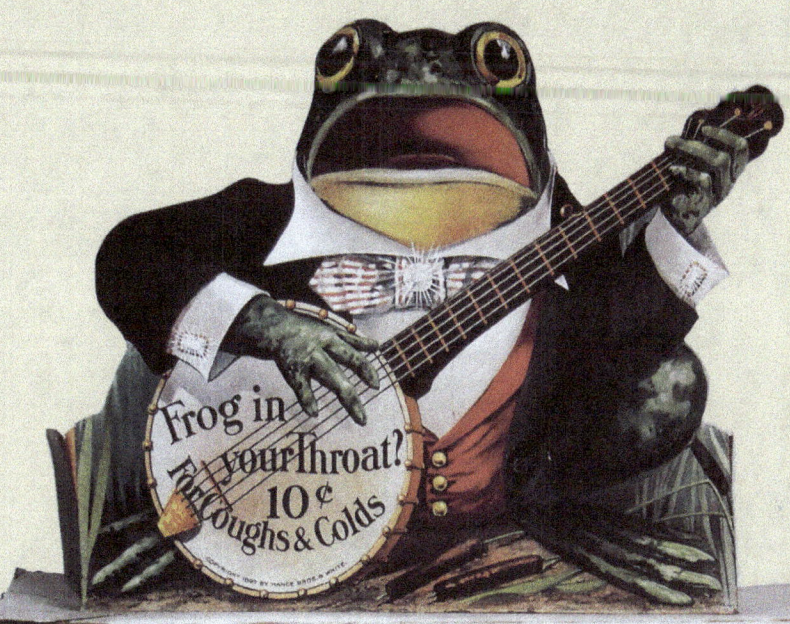

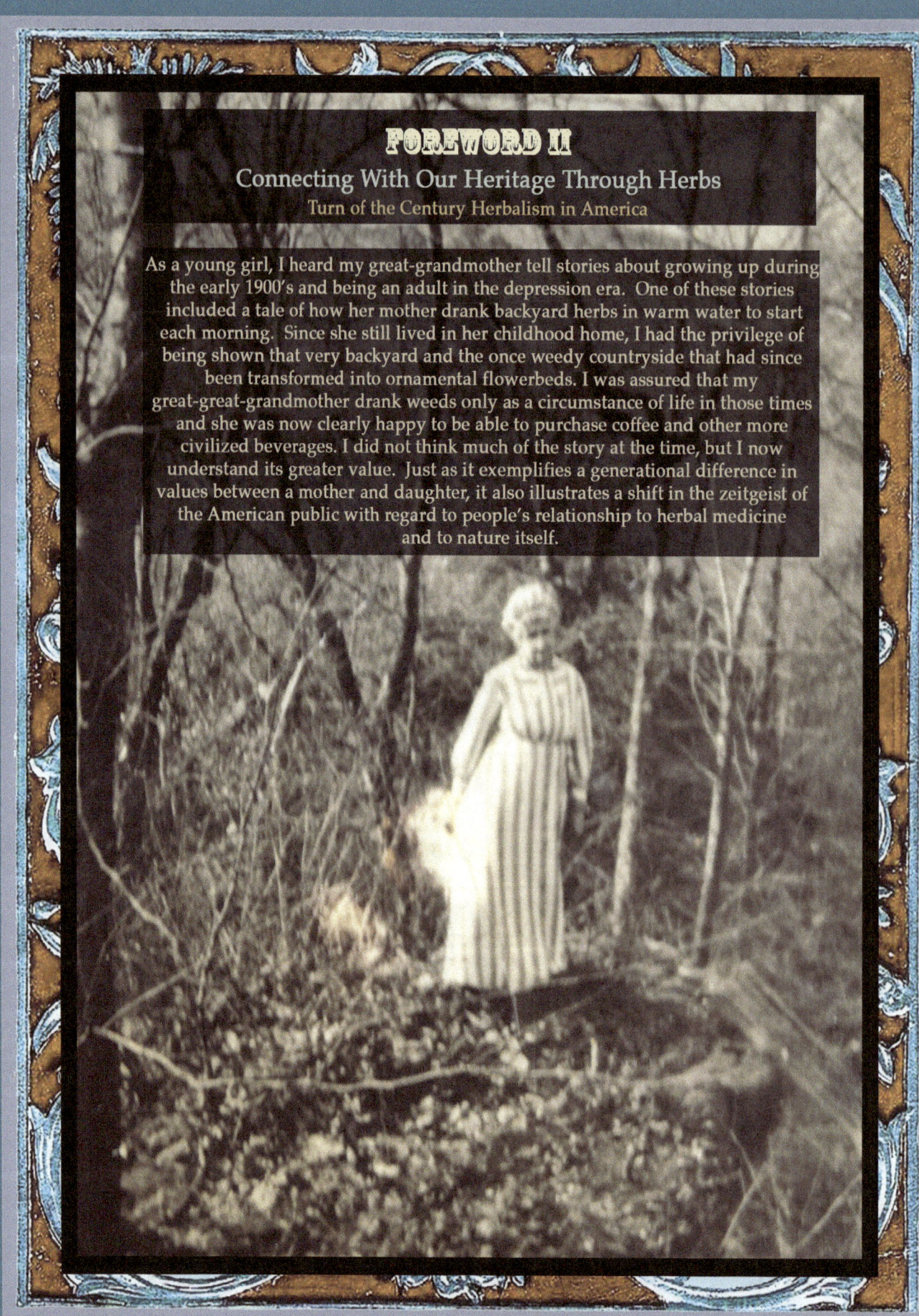

# FOREWORD II
## Connecting With Our Heritage Through Herbs
### Turn of the Century Herbalism in America

As a young girl, I heard my great-grandmother tell stories about growing up during the early 1900's and being an adult in the depression era. One of these stories included a tale of how her mother drank backyard herbs in warm water to start each morning. Since she still lived in her childhood home, I had the privilege of being shown that very backyard and the once weedy countryside that had since been transformed into ornamental flowerbeds. I was assured that my great-great-grandmother drank weeds only as a circumstance of life in those times and she was now clearly happy to be able to purchase coffee and other more civilized beverages. I did not think much of the story at the time, but I now understand its greater value. Just as it exemplifies a generational difference in values between a mother and daughter, it also illustrates a shift in the zeitgeist of the American public with regard to people's relationship to herbal medicine and to nature itself.

A connection to herbs, nature, and self-reliance in personal healthcare was part of life for most folks until well into the 20th century. Attitudes started to change when the 1906 Pure Food and Drug Act began to expose some products' exaggerated claims of "curing" all varieties of aliments and serious illnesses. This began to sow the seeds of doubt in consumers' minds and by the 1930's corporate advertising slogans such as DuPont's "Better things for better living through chemistry" were penetrating people's minds everywhere.

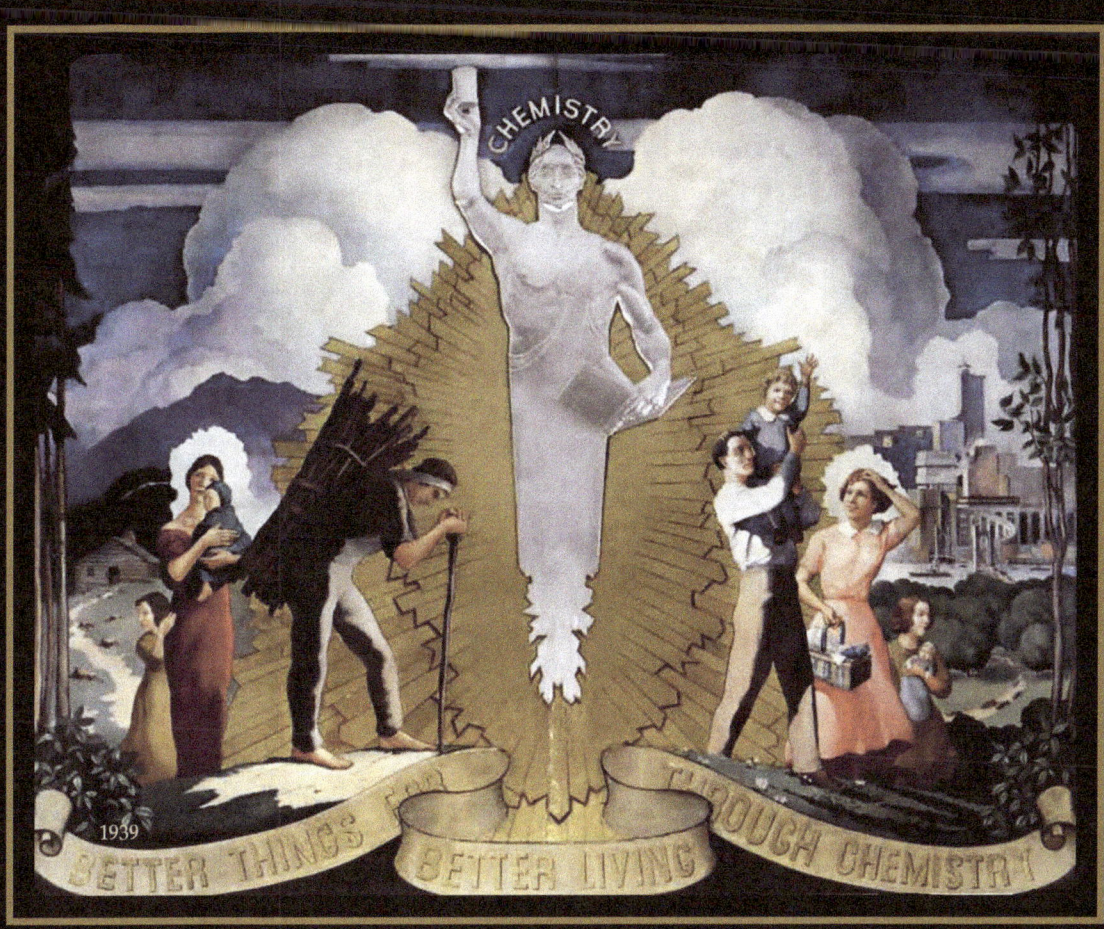

This shift in public thinking gained further momentum in the 1940s when mass production of modern laboratory medicines, beginning with Penicillin, further undermined people's faith in herbs and weakened their connection to the natural world. Advertisements such as this one from pharmaceutical company Eli Lilly appeared in a 1944 pharmacists' journal and would influence America's prevailing attitude toward herbalism:

*The 'medicine man' of the early nineteen hundreds has small part in our modern habits of living. Little medicine is sold these days from the tailboard of a wagon… A reputation for cheapness in prescription merchandise is despised by everyone. The Lilly label identifies you as a competent prescriptionist."*

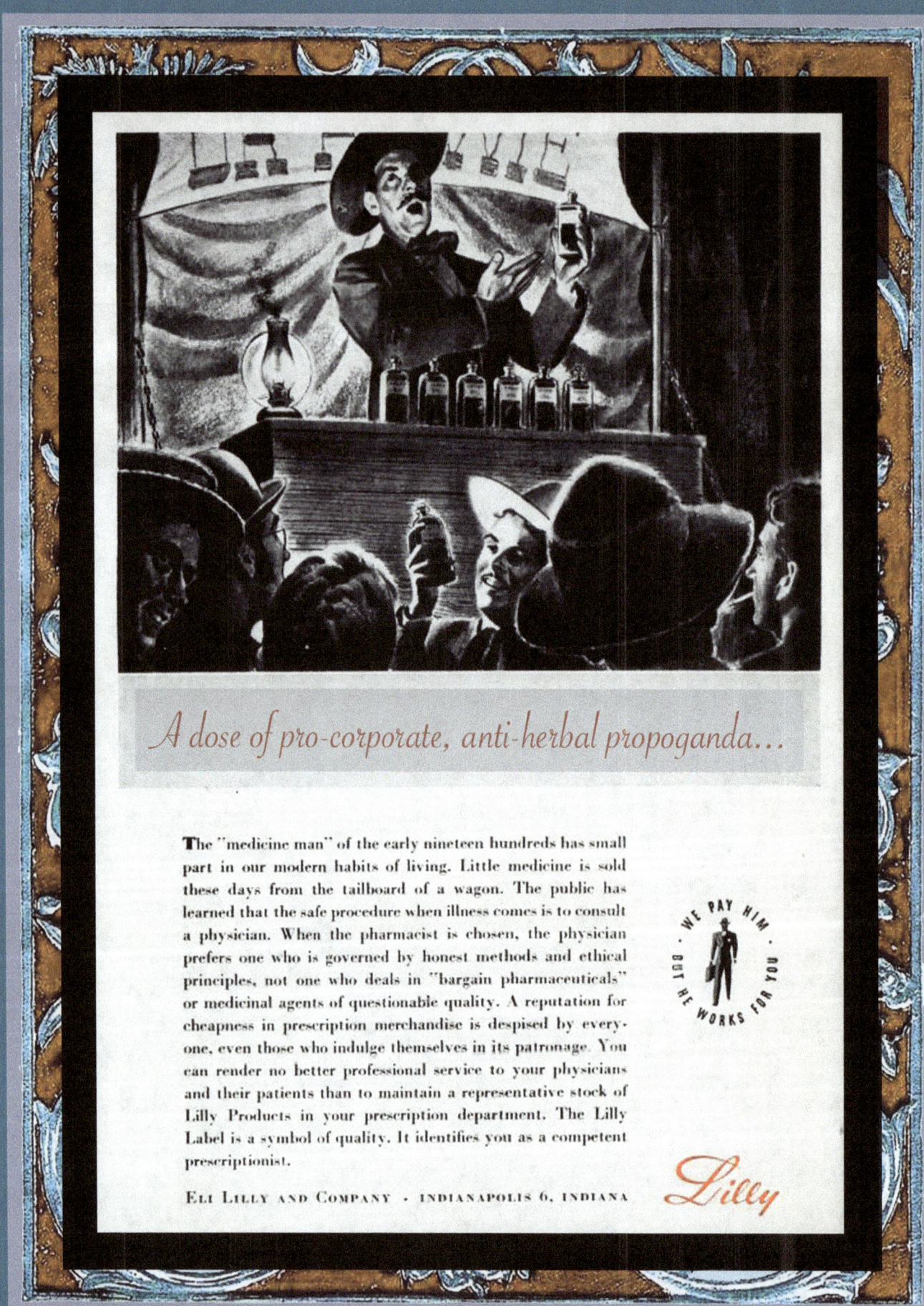

From the 1880s and into the early 1900s, the Mother Gray Company of Le Roy New York made a number of popular herbal remedies including Allen's Foot Ease and Mother Gray's Sweet Worm Powders. Products made prior to the 1906 Pure Food and Drug Act were not required to list ingredients and often made sweeping cure-all claims such as those on the box of Mother Gray's Australian Leaf tea blend. The box states "a certain cure for headache, backache, bearing down pains, kidney, liver, bladder, and urinary troubles, diabetes, and dropsy". The package further states, "it cures female weakness including inflammation and ulceration, irregular and painful or suppressed illness and all diseases of the stomach, bowels and urinary organs in either sex". No ingredients are listed, which makes it is impossible to know how many of these conditions might have been affected by the formula. Regardless of ingredients, any claims of curing so many ailments in a single remedy should naturally raise suspicions. These exaggerated claims would provide a foundation for federal regulation and a catalyst for the shift in beliefs about herbal remedies that would unfold during the coming years.

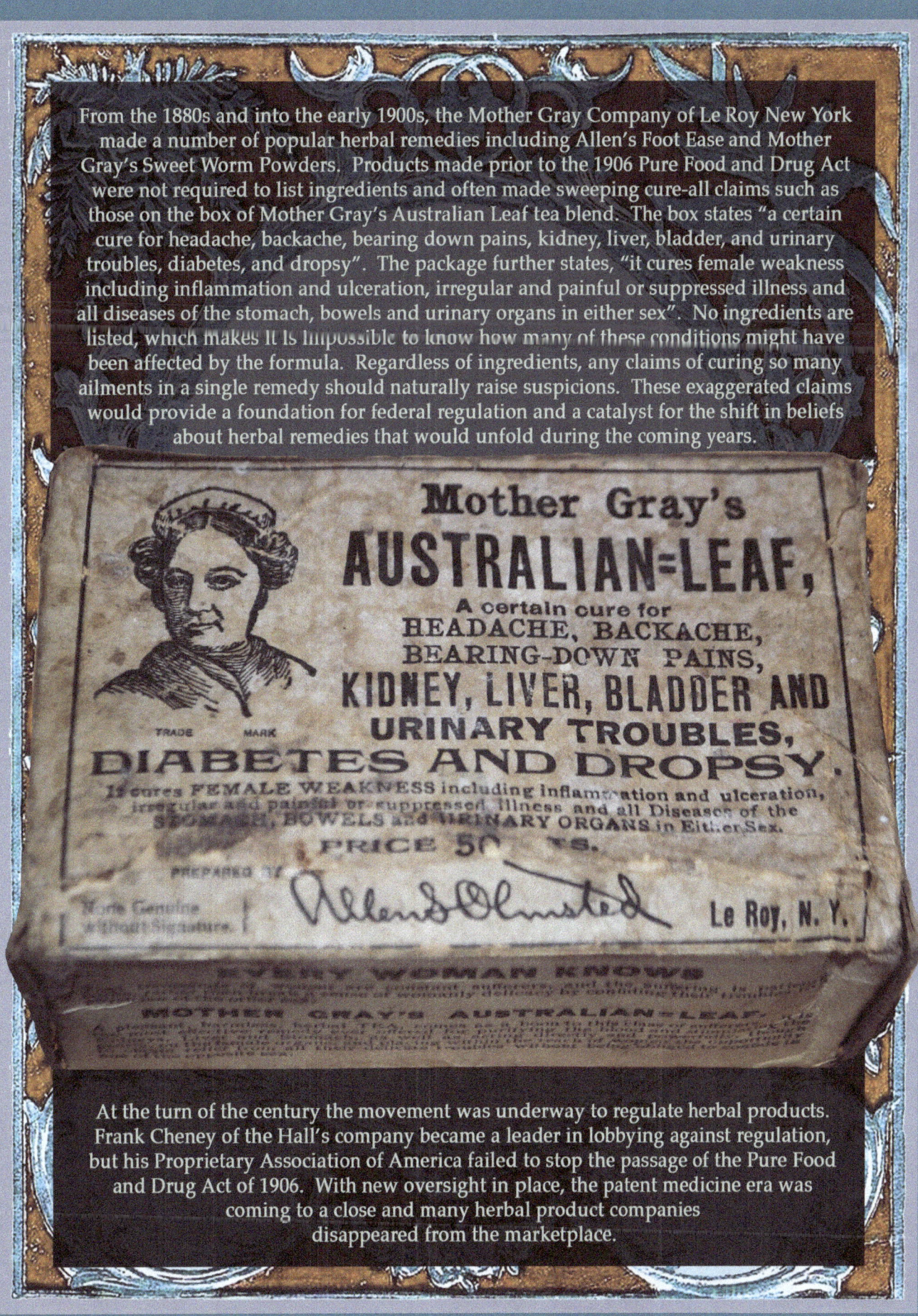

At the turn of the century the movement was underway to regulate herbal products. Frank Cheney of the Hall's company became a leader in lobbying against regulation, but his Proprietary Association of America failed to stop the passage of the Pure Food and Drug Act of 1906. With new oversight in place, the patent medicine era was coming to a close and many herbal product companies disappeared from the marketplace.

As a result of the new regulations, the surviving companies increased newspaper adverting. The Hall's company ran ads in newspapers across the country offering $100 to anyone who could produce catarrh that could not be remedied by his popular product Hall's Catarrh Cure. Another result was that companies such as Hall's, Romero Drug, Los Angels Pharmacal, and Dr. J. H. McLean's Medicine all began listing ingredients on their remedies and the outlandish cure-all claims disappeared from packaging.

Upon inspection of the ingredients, we can see more clearly the continuation of our herbal heritage. Many of these products contain the same herbs we might use today for the same purposes. Liniments such as Aztec, La Sanadora, and McLean's Volcanic Oil were made with Cayenne, Menthol, Pine, and Camphor to ease the sore muscles of everyday life. Halls' syrup included honey and zinc to ease sore throats associated with colds. Essence of Peppermint was a popular staple of any home apothecary and was used for all manner of ailments, just as it is today.

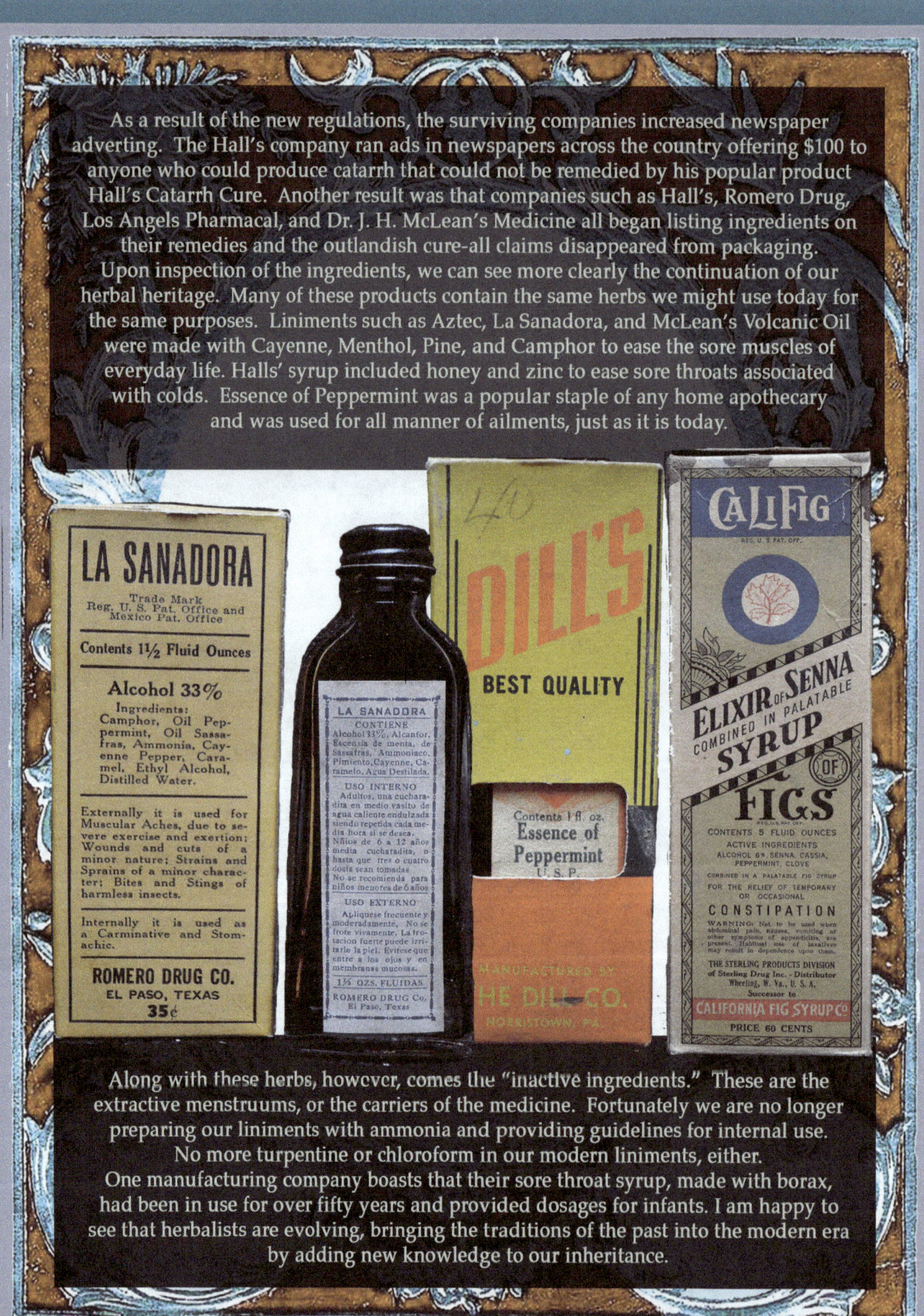

Along with these herbs, however, comes the "inactive ingredients." These are the extractive menstruums, or the carriers of the medicine. Fortunately we are no longer preparing our liniments with ammonia and providing guidelines for internal use. No more turpentine or chloroform in our modern liniments, either.

One manufacturing company boasts that their sore throat syrup, made with borax, had been in use for over fifty years and provided dosages for infants. I am happy to see that herbalists are evolving, bringing the traditions of the past into the modern era by adding new knowledge to our inheritance.

Later products of the 1930s and 40s illuminate the continuing importance of herbal products in the lives of Americans during and after the Great Depression, but also act as harbingers of coming change. This was a time of economic hardship when many people could not afford physician's fees and self-care skills continued to be of great value. Remedies including Argotane, Bukets, and Califig still used herbal terms on their labels such as tonic, cholagogue, and elixir or phrases such as "stimulant to the diuretic action of the kidneys". Some products like Sterling Drug's Califig syrup continued on in the traditions of the past by offering an herbal remedy containing Senna, Cassia, Cloves, and Peppermint for the treatment of constipation. However, businesses such as the Argotano Company (a division of Plough Inc.) were bridging the past and future with new formulas and promotional tactics. Argotane frequently ran ads in newspapers across the country extolling the virtues of their product. These ads were disguised as news articles with titles and subtitles such as "Mrs. Hays One of the Proudest Women in Amarillo, Texas, I'm Certainly Grateful For the Happiness Arogtane Has Brought Home."

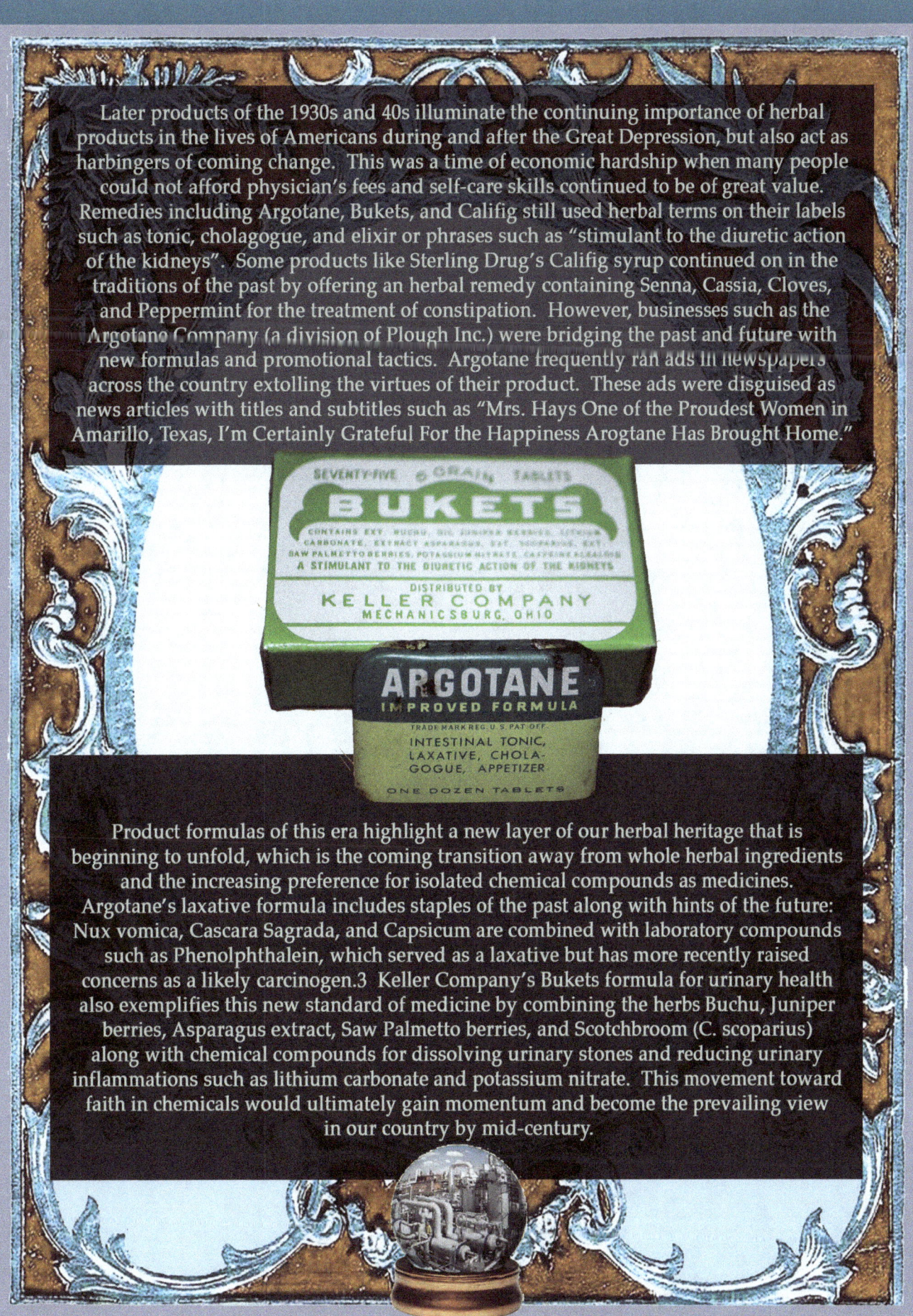

Product formulas of this era highlight a new layer of our herbal heritage that is beginning to unfold, which is the coming transition away from whole herbal ingredients and the increasing preference for isolated chemical compounds as medicines. Argotane's laxative formula includes staples of the past along with hints of the future: Nux vomica, Cascara Sagrada, and Capsicum are combined with laboratory compounds such as Phenolphthalein, which served as a laxative but has more recently raised concerns as a likely carcinogen.[3] Keller Company's Bukets formula for urinary health also exemplifies this new standard of medicine by combining the herbs Buchu, Juniper berries, Asparagus extract, Saw Palmetto berries, and Scotchbroom (C. scoparius) along with chemical compounds for dissolving urinary stones and reducing urinary inflammations such as lithium carbonate and potassium nitrate. This movement toward faith in chemicals would ultimately gain momentum and become the prevailing view in our country by mid-century.

These are some of the layers of our rich and diverse herbal heritage. The shift in the American public's relationship to herbal remedies is exemplified through my great-grandmother's story about her mother. In one generation a new attitude was clearly emerging about herbalism. Prior to the turn of the 20th century, weeds and common plants were what people turned to when health issues came up or they were simply added to the diet as a source of reliable and affordable nutrition. This was a time of westward expansion, settling new territories, and carving out an existence in new and sometimes hostile environments. It was also an era when people spent time outdoors, lived off the land, and made household items by hand. During this time and continuing on through the Depression era we can clearly see the common threads connecting our modern herbal practice to that of our predecessors through an examination of popular herbal formulas. As the 1900s rolled on and industrialized modernity settled in, people gradually began to view herbs as an inferior remedy of the past with new 'scientific' drugs marketed by powerful pharmaceutical companies to take their place. Now that we have experienced over half a century of 'better living through chemicals' many of us are beginning to seek a more balanced view to life. Wilderness is no longer something to be tamed and conquered, but something to protect and relish. The movement is well underway to circle back around to self-reliance in personal healthcare through natural medicines. This is likely influenced by various factors including the preventive vaccination regime and antibiotic 'safety-net' that modern medicine has provided as well as the decrease in frightening acute illnesses and the rise of chronic inflammatory illnesses. (Ironically, the shift from acute to chronic ailments may be precipitated, in part, by the pervasive use of chemicals in our lives.) While herbal medicine in post industrialized America is usually lumped into the category known as "alternative medicine", many of us know that it is actually traditional medicine, and the original *medicine of the people.*

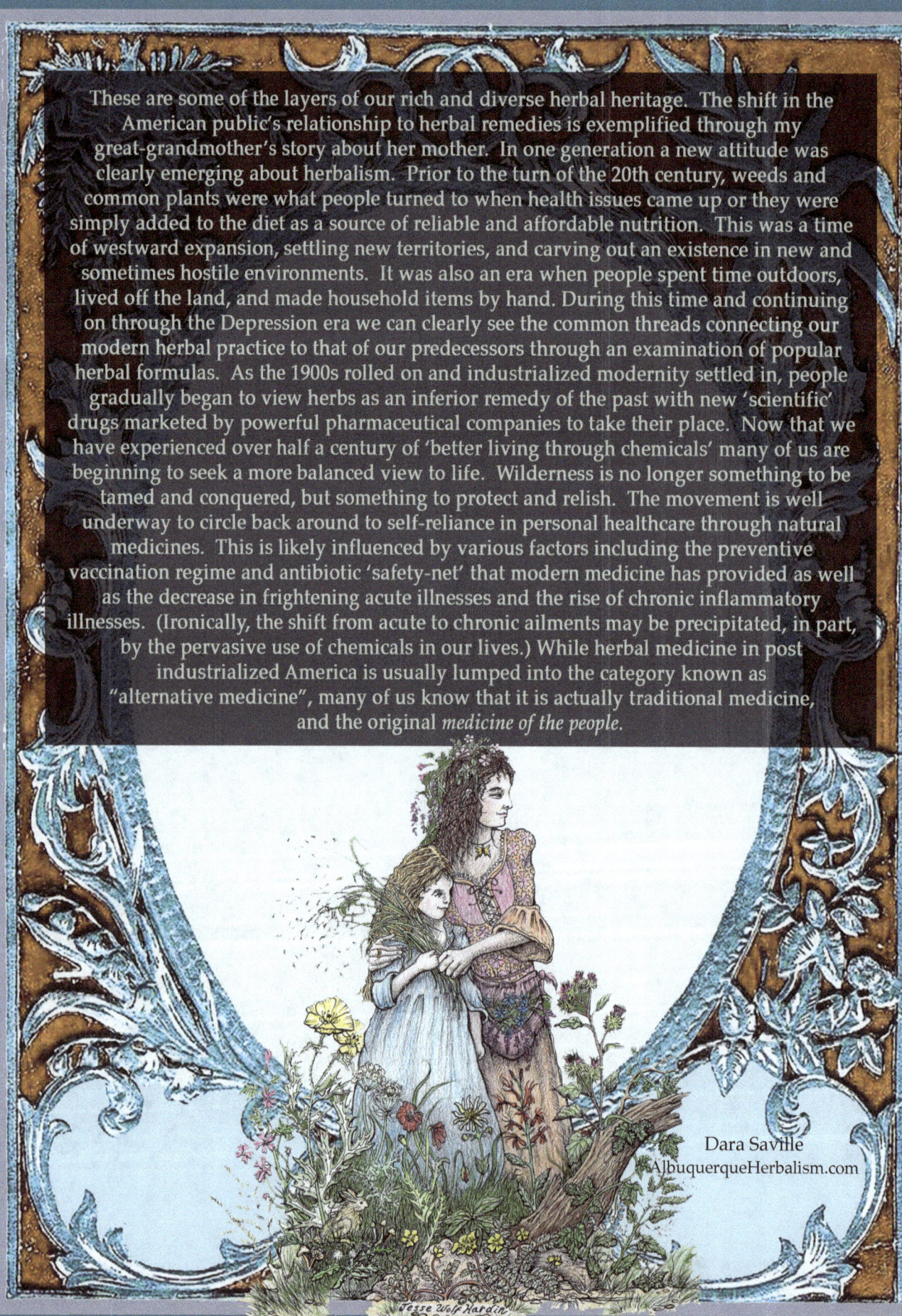

Dara Saville
AlbuquerqueHerbalism.com

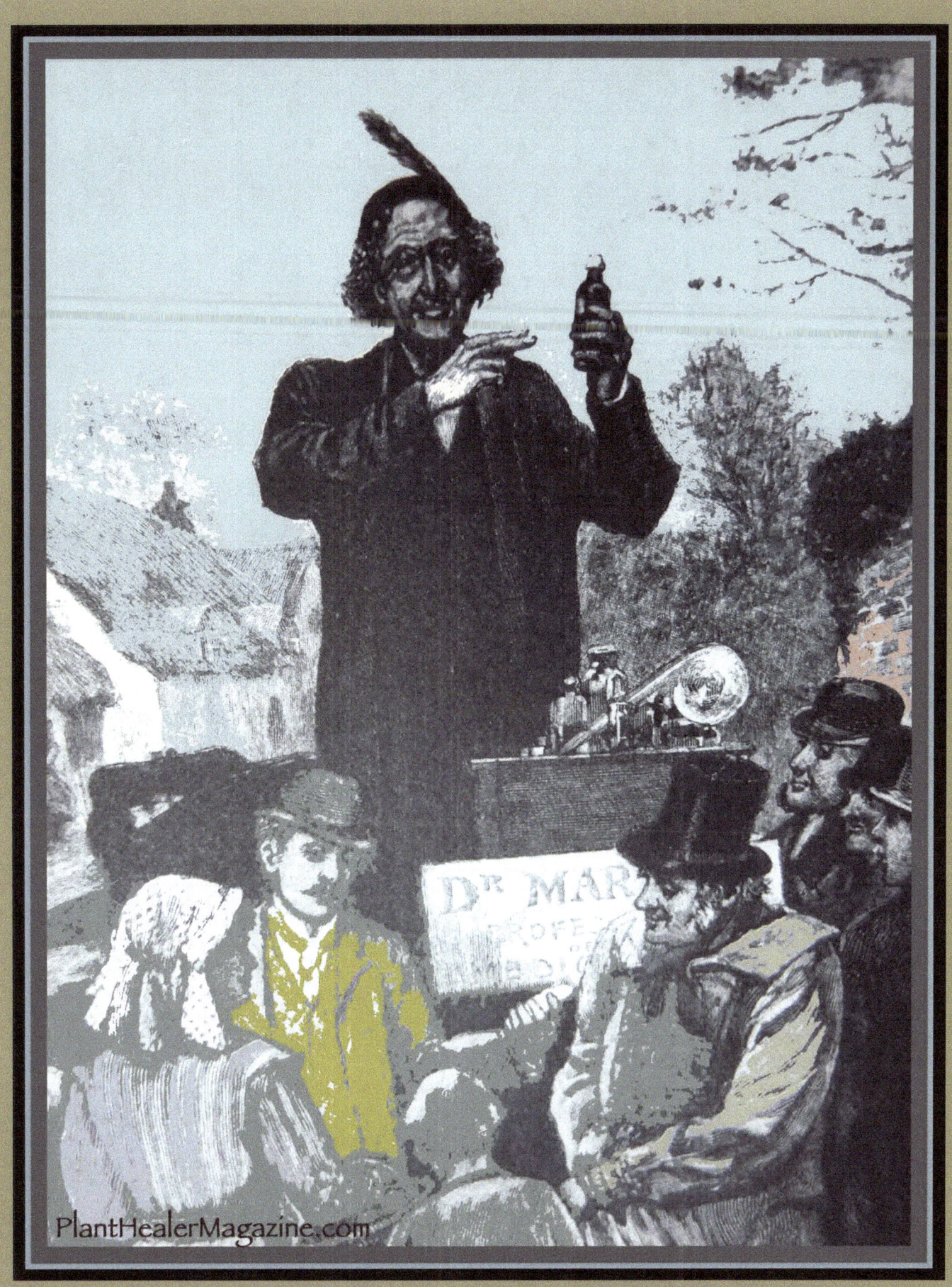

# Act I

## ON THE MEDICINE TRAIL
### Herbs & Entertainment for The Common Folk

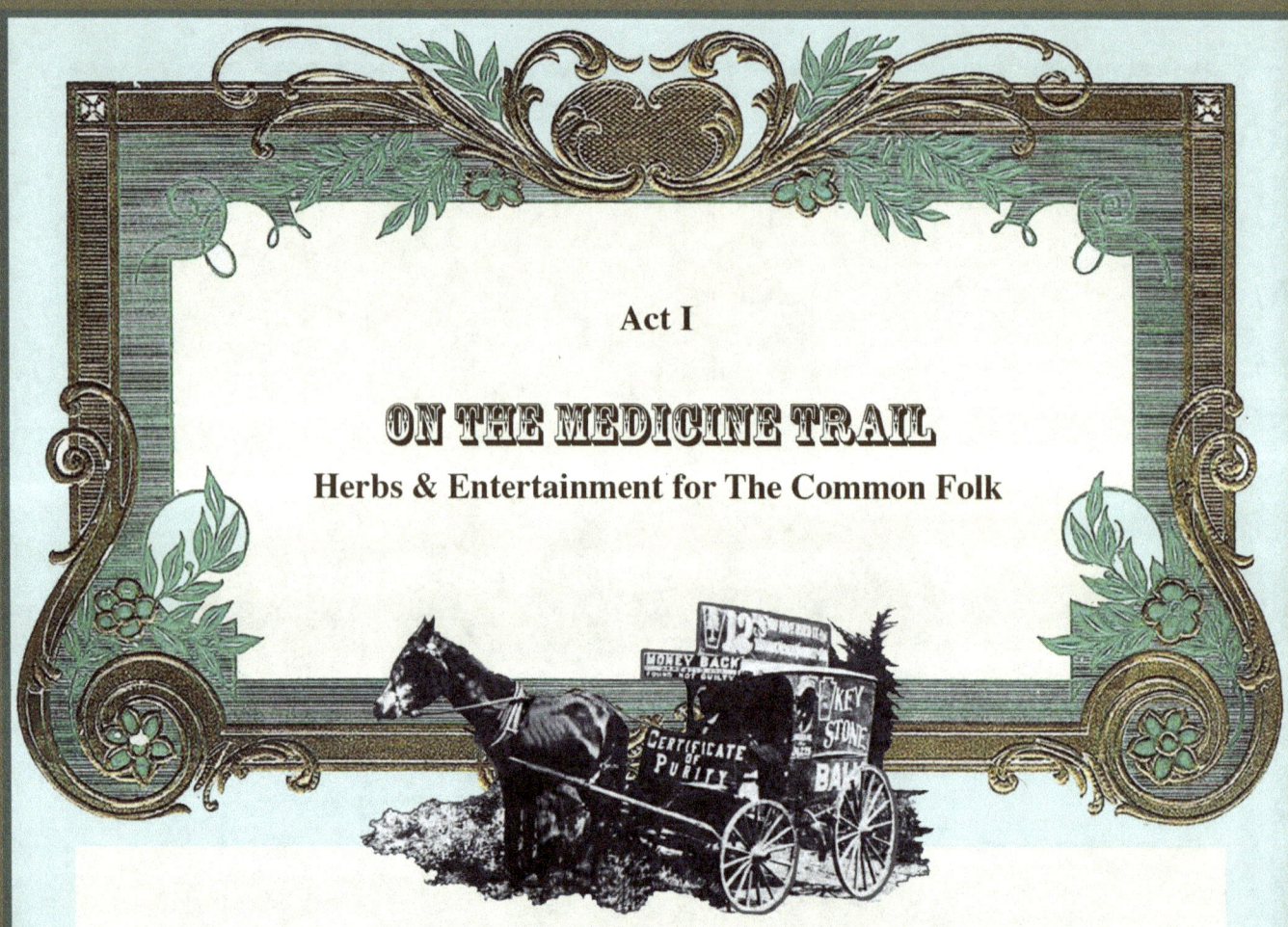

*"I was born in the wagon of a travelin' show, mother used to dance for the money they'd throw. Father would do whatever he could, preach a little gospel, sell a couple bottles of Doctor Goode's."*
–Cher (Gypsies, Tramps & Thieves)

Imagine if you will, an incidence of herbal edification and hungered-for entertainment that would repeat itself again and again all across rural America. The site might be a town square, a popular dusty crossroads, the speaker's platform at a "newfangled" air show park or simply a local farmer's unplowed field. Except for any differences in vegetation and topography, it could just as well be located anywhere from northern Georgia to western Pennsylvania, the gold fields of California or the farmlands of the Great Plains, always far from the big cities and in places where people lived close to the land. Corn shuckers and melon growers, home-canners and cowboys. It has a timeless feel, and could be anytime from the end of the Civil War until the 1930s. While cities swelled and were electrified, popular fashions evolved and government centralized, the site we picture will have changed relatively little in 50 years, with seed company advertisements fading from the sides of barns, barefoot boys chewing on long grass stems while kicking cans down the railroad tracks stretching beyond our sight. Livestock mill about close by, as stacks of hay summon generations of young lovers to spoon and play. The people you see are a hardy breed quick to speak up about the importance of self reliance and self sufficiency, whether they speak with mountainous Colorado inflections or an Alabama front-porch drawl. Most of them repair their own clothes until they'll no longer hold together, and their labors often produce enough food for their entire families to eat. Many of them know about the medicinal plants that grow wildly in the area, and all tend to see self-healthcare as not just a necessity but as an individual responsibility and a natural-given right.

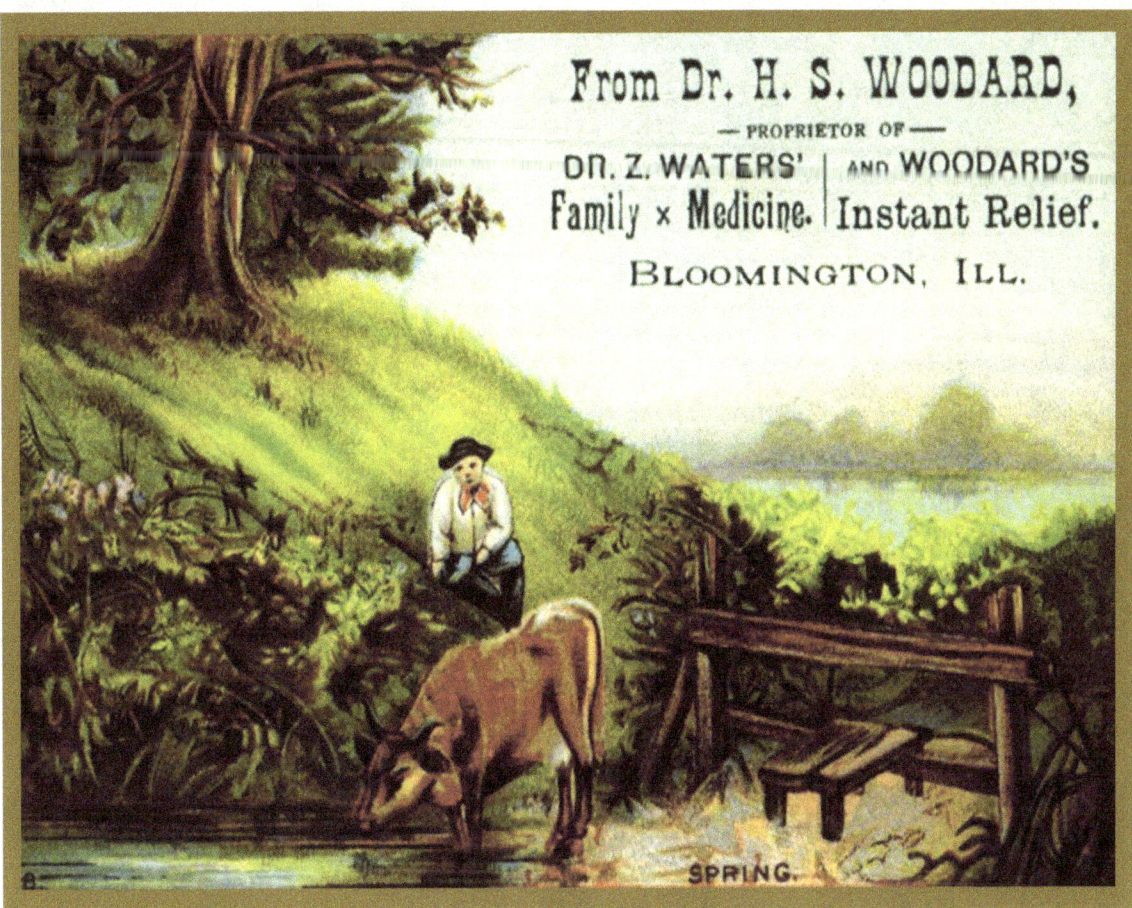

Entertainment around these parts would usually amount to no more than a family or two getting together for an evening of contra dancing or the neighborhood women getting out their thimbles and needles for a Saturday sewing-bee. Folks would be happy for almost any diversion from the regularity of small town regimens and monotony of daily farm chores, stopping what they were doing just to ogle a stranger passing through, or to make bets on the expected failure or success of a gopher-huntin' dog. Nearly everyone from miles around would turn out at first wind of the arrival of a traveling circus troupe, political stump speech or banjo driven minstrel show, and it didn't matter what their spiritual persuasion when there came a chance to participate in an evangelical revival in a tent hastily set up for the purpose.

The horses are pulled to a stop at a prearranged spot or anywhere that looks likely to get a good draw, released from their harnesses and tied by ropes and halters to a nearby tree. Stepping smartly down from the driver's seat – or rising with a flourish from within the oakwood coach –will be a man dressed at least a tad more flamboyantly than the overalls-clad fellows lined up to meet him with their mouths open and hands in their pants. Doffing a snappy bowler, Stetson or silken top hat, he clears the road grunge from his throat, then loudly introduces himself and his mission to the growing throng."Well," he might begin, "a fine afternoon to all you gentleman of good will and ladies of fine tastes! It is I, the man known as the people's physician, maestro of popular music and entertainment, your alchemist of well being and conveyor of necessary remedies for a well balanced and fruitful life... asking you each but a single question: What, dear friends, is the price of health?

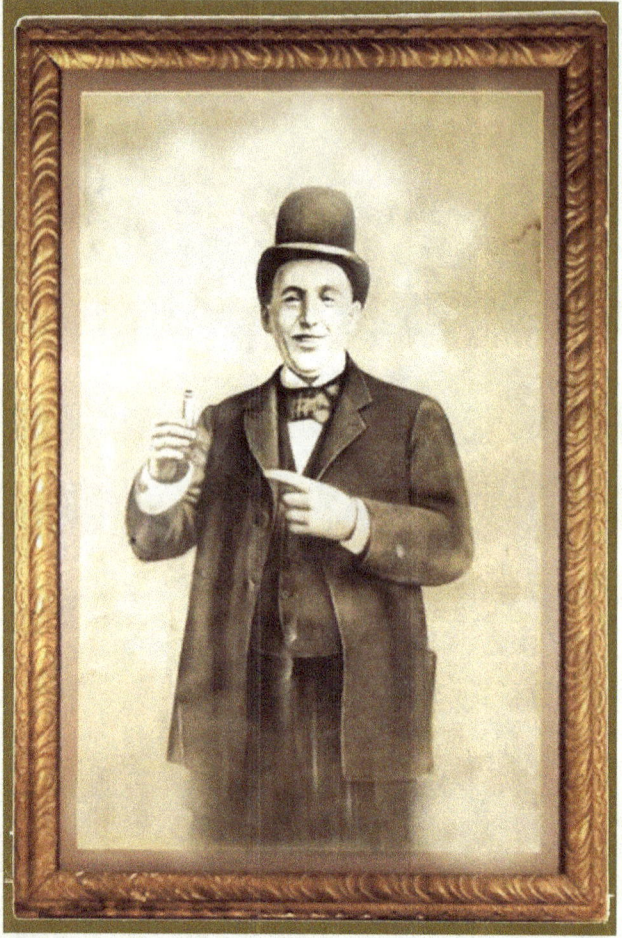

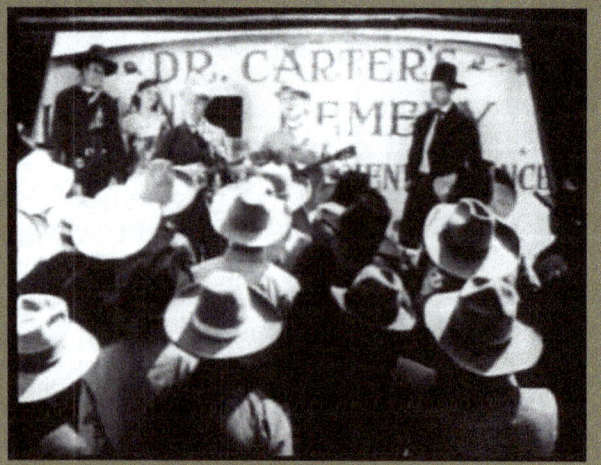

"For a mere fifty pennies gathering dust in your bureau drawer, two measly quarters or five thin dimes, you too can avail yourselves of nature's own medicines, for what overpriced doctor could ever know more or do more for us than Mother Nature herself? As God has given to us all manner of plants to feed our bellies and heal our wounds and infirmities, I have been given the secrets of their use by his agents living closest to his creation. But wait!"

"I am not here simply to treat your maladies but to ease your burdens and help raise your spirits. Before I have dispensed a single bottle of my herbal preparations, I shall have first dispensed a humble display of well practiced magic and the pleasures of song."

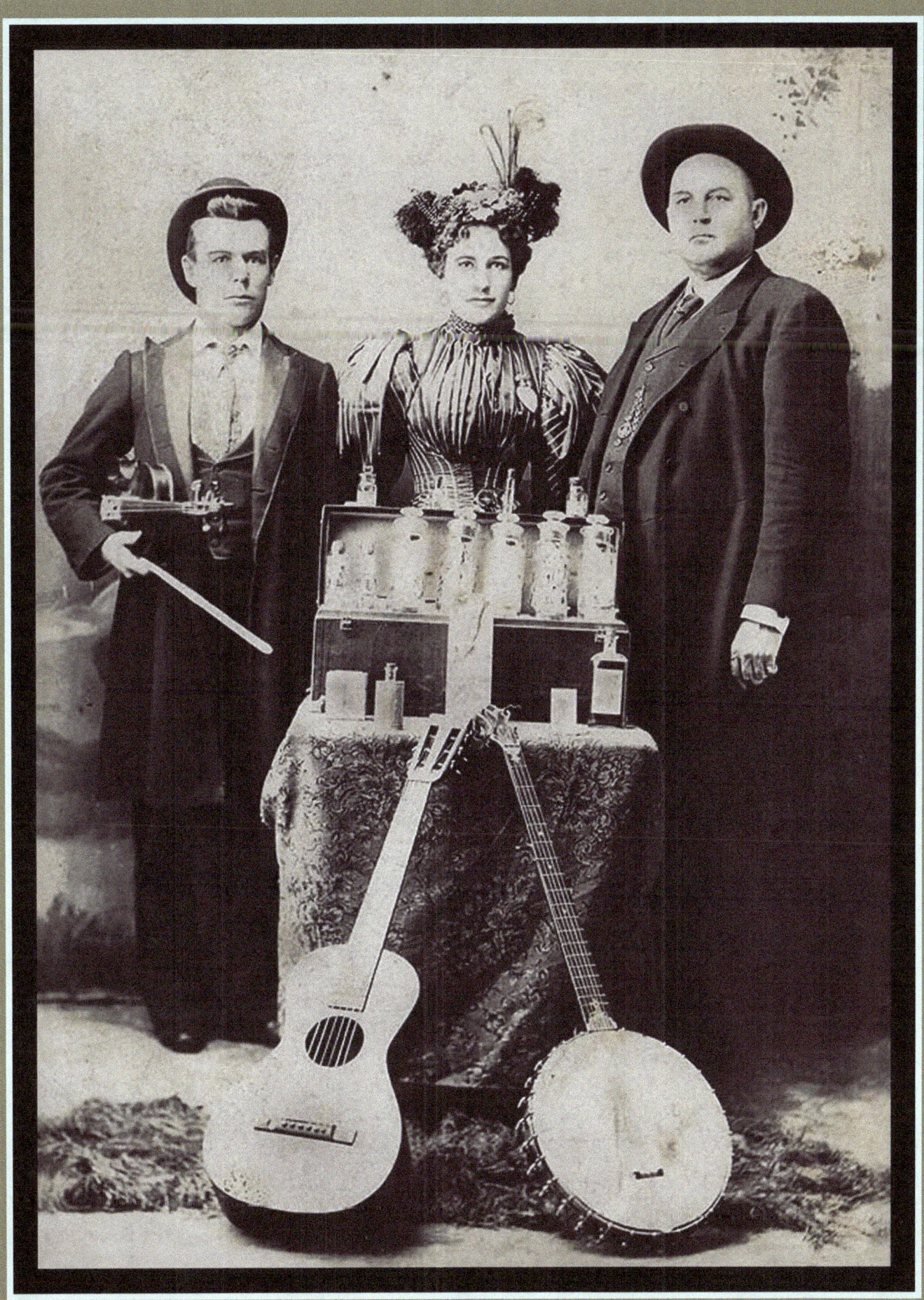

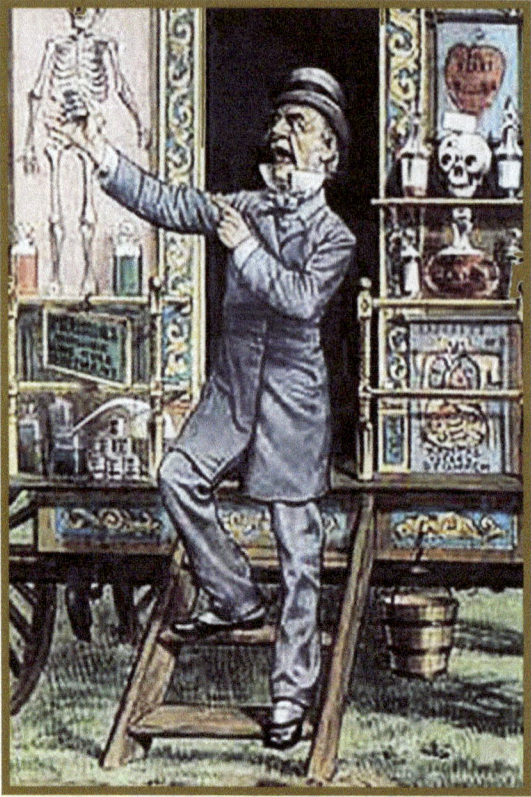

If he has assistants or performers to help, they will have soon set up the visual attractions – from anatomy charts and pressed plants to human skulls and exotic butterfly collections, shrunken heads purportedly from New Guinea and even floral mosaics made up of the teeth extracted from a succession of willing audiences. Sometimes called "the museum," these exhibitions did indeed constitute traveling museums for the rural working class and the poor in an age when visitors to most urban collections were largely limited to the rich and privileged. Such displays were sources of education and delight, as much as magnets attracting people to the products and shows.

The importance of these shows to any who attended should not be underestimated. For many, it would be their first exposure to various kinds of music including compositions from disparate cultures from around the world.

While the banjo and guitar were commonplace enough, there were also harmoniums and accordions, savage rhythmic drums and flutes played by turban-wearing musicians from old Bombay, clapping gospel singers, and wild-eyed violinists laying down melodies for the propulsion and transport of modestly veiled belly dancers. Like the minstrel shows that preceded them, the Medicine Shows afforded people in out of the way places the experience of being a part of larger human family, and before the advent of radio became one of the main means for the spreading of new and popular songs. Many a singer got their start on the road, writing new tunes to the clinking and jingling of road jostled tincture bottles.

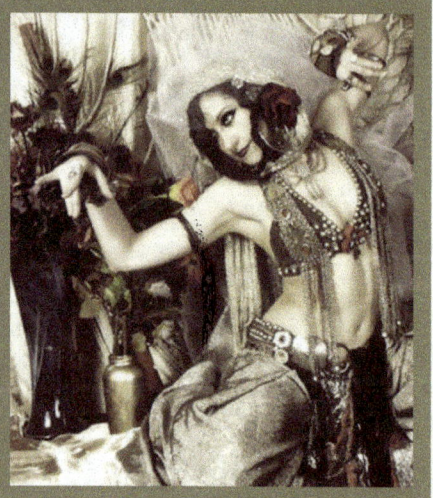

As late as the 1940s the Medicine Show-inspired Hadacol Caravan trains were featuring performers like Hank Williams and Roy Acuff. The earlier, smaller shows were often well loved for providing such entertaining "ballyhoo."

"You," says the Medicine Man, "can purchase a bottle for what ails ya later... be it some tincture or tea, but the pleasures of the night *are free, free, free!*"

The success of the Medicine Show "pitchman" hinged in part on the quality of his spiel, known as "the pitch" or "the give." As the "grinder" Fred "Doc" Bloodgood put it, "I have always made it my practice never to use one word where four will do." Then again, not all were said to have a way with words. Some were "boozer" doctors who muddled their sentences whenever "in the cups," a few like Indian John muttered rapid biblical verse scarcely intelligible yet somehow sufficiently impressive, while others chose to let their medicines or their banjos do the talking.

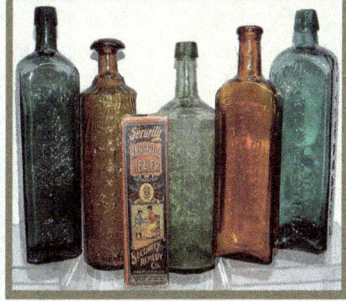

The message in every case was a very Jacksonian one: doctors could barely be afforded and seldom trusted, the most natural medicines are the best; the means to ease suffering and illness should be equally available to all; and we need to empower ourselves to make our own medical choices, to take responsibility for ours and our family's health needs,

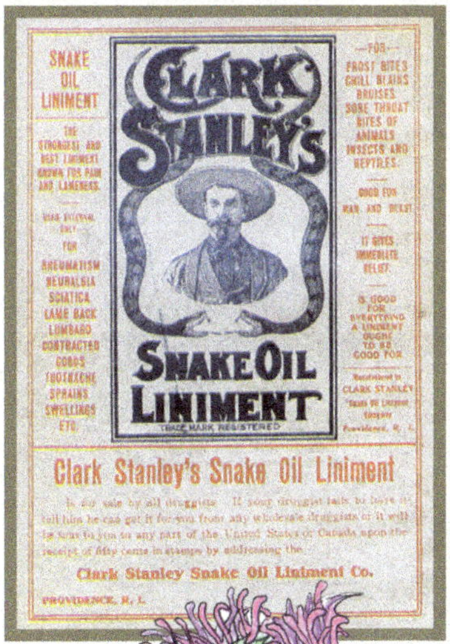

Some Medicine Men were hucksters for sure, but the bottom line is that few of these traveling pitchmen and their home brewed tonics and tinctures did nowhere near as much harm as the licensed doctors, iffy treatments and commercial pills and capsules of their day, and a majority provided genuinely effective herbal relief to the rural, the impoverished, and the marginalized folks of America. Yet, they found themselves under attack by what were the true "patent medicine" sellers: the swelling pharmaceutical companies harking their synthetic wares, eager to see the nation's easily obtained plant medicines supplanted by their expensive menu of drugs. No wonder that all herbal sellers, not just the charlatans and scam artists – were publicly vilified in magazines and newspapers, with such a determined campaign launched to destroy them!

It is no wonder, as well, that today's informed practitioners of herbalism and natural healing have begun learning to embrace the Traveling Medicine Show tradition, as a dramatic and inspiring chapter in a long and winding history – the rolling roots of the archetypal Medicine Wagon, and the individual medicine trails that we each still travel.

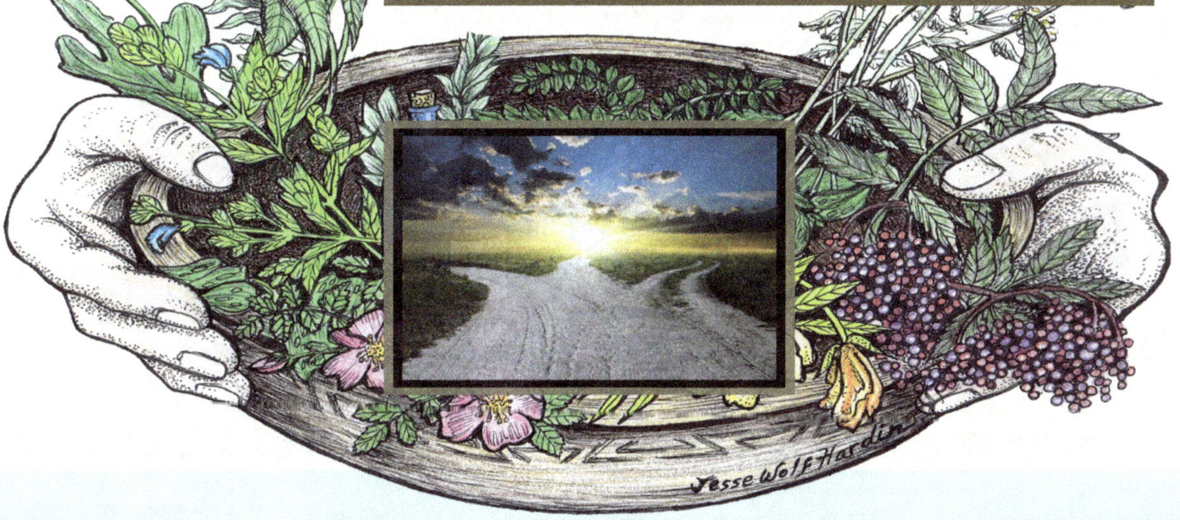

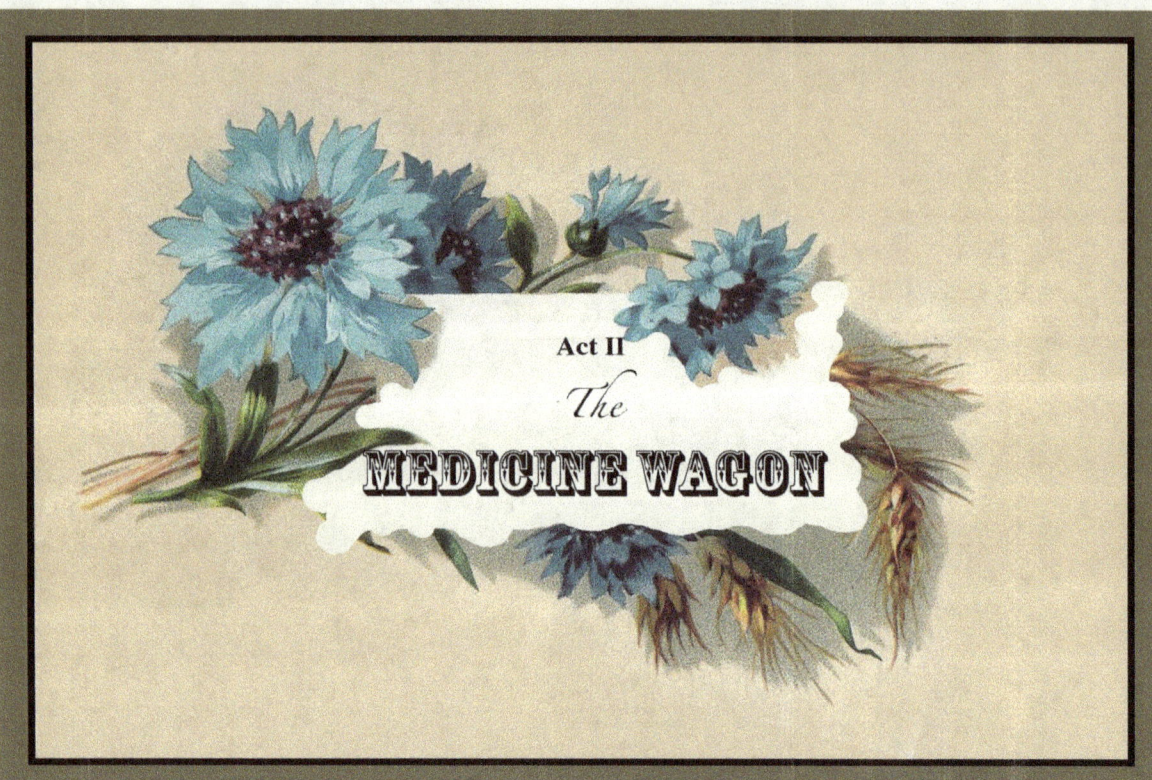

Act II

# The MEDICINE WAGON

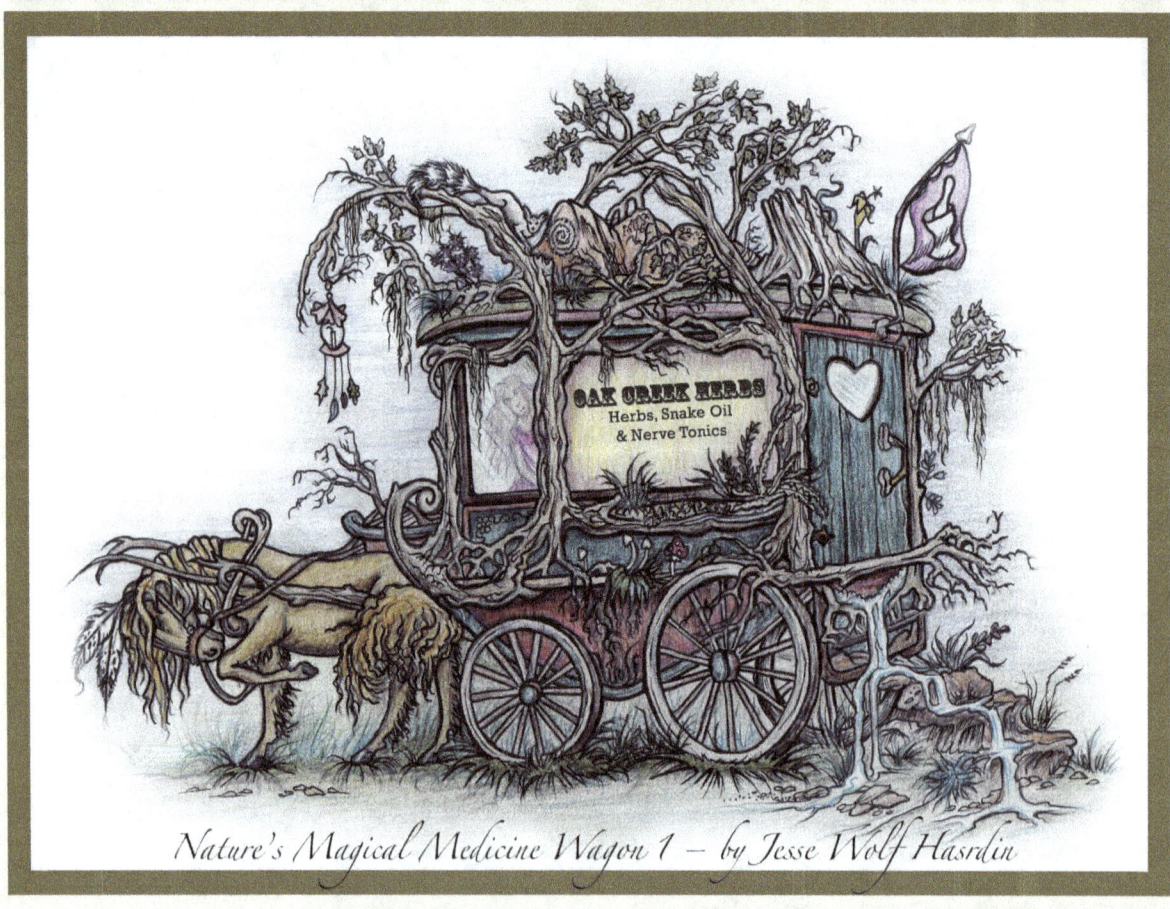

*Nature's Magical Medicine Wagon 1 — by Jesse Wolf Hasrdin*

There could have been no Traveling Medicine Shows without the proverbial Medicine Wagon.
What a medicine seller needed on the circuit was a safe way to transport his precious cargo – herbal concoctions that took weeks to make and bottle, necessarily stored in fragile glass.
The earliest wagons were horse-drawn of course, over the seldom repaired roads that lead into the rural hinterlands, the simplest of these being no more than an open topped buckboard.

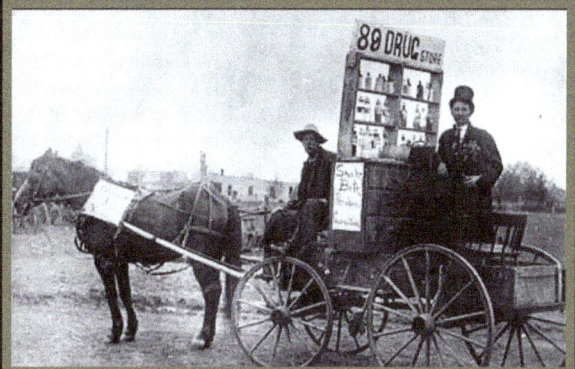

The most elaborate and purposed to the trade were the custom enclosed wagons designed to be slept in as well to carry the goods, and those limited edition salesman's models where the entire wagon was filled with wooden cabinets and drawers, each compartment lined and padded to decrease the chances of breakage.

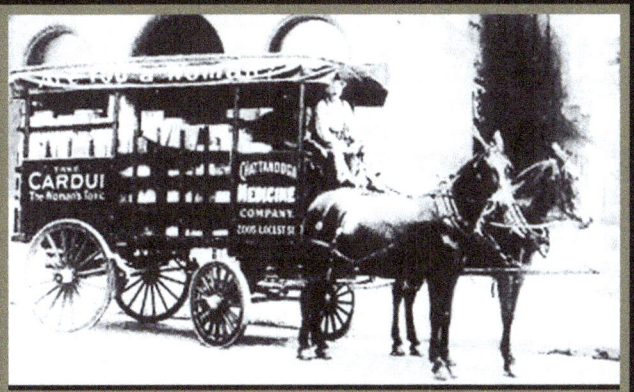 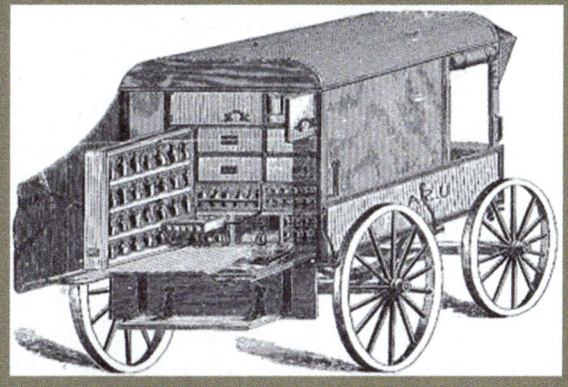

It must be remembered that the majority of "shows" were no more than speeches given by a single Medicine Man as he stood next to his wagon of healthful wares on the streets of each out-of-the-way town he visited, and a much more basic and inexpensive buggy was sufficient.
Some sellers even made their rounds on horseback, as indicated by the medicine "panniers" constructed for carry atop one's favorite gelding or mare.

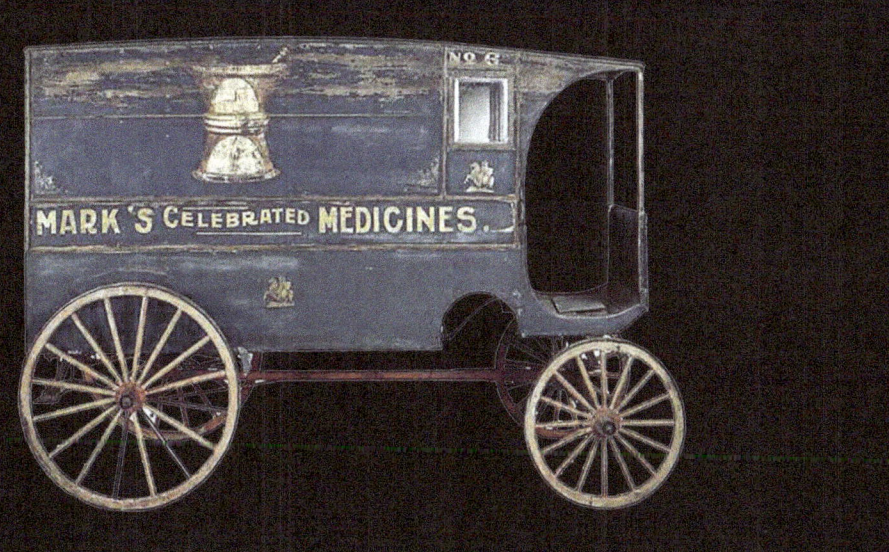

2  ADVERTISEMENTS.

# THE BEST
# SADDLE BAG
## IN THE MARKET.

ELLIOTT'S PATENT SADDLE BAG

**IT HAS NO DRAWERS.**
It is Made of one Piece.

**NICKEL PLATED FINISHINGS.**
No Seams or Stitches.

### READ THE FOLLOWING INDORSEMENT.

"I write to say that I am more than pleased with the Elliott's Patent Medical Saddle Bags, and I have used them sufficiently long to give me a very high appreciation of their compactness, lightness, and convenience of arrangement. These advantages they present in an eminent degree over the styles generally in use. Physicians in country and town practice will find them useful and invaluable. I remain, very respectfully,
Your obedient servant,     A. M. FAUNTLEROY, M. D.
Ex-President Medical Society of Va.

**MORE ELLIOTT'S PATENT ARE SOLD THAN ALL OTHERS COMBINED.
ADOPTED BY THE U. S. GOVERNMENT OVER ALL COMPETITORS.**

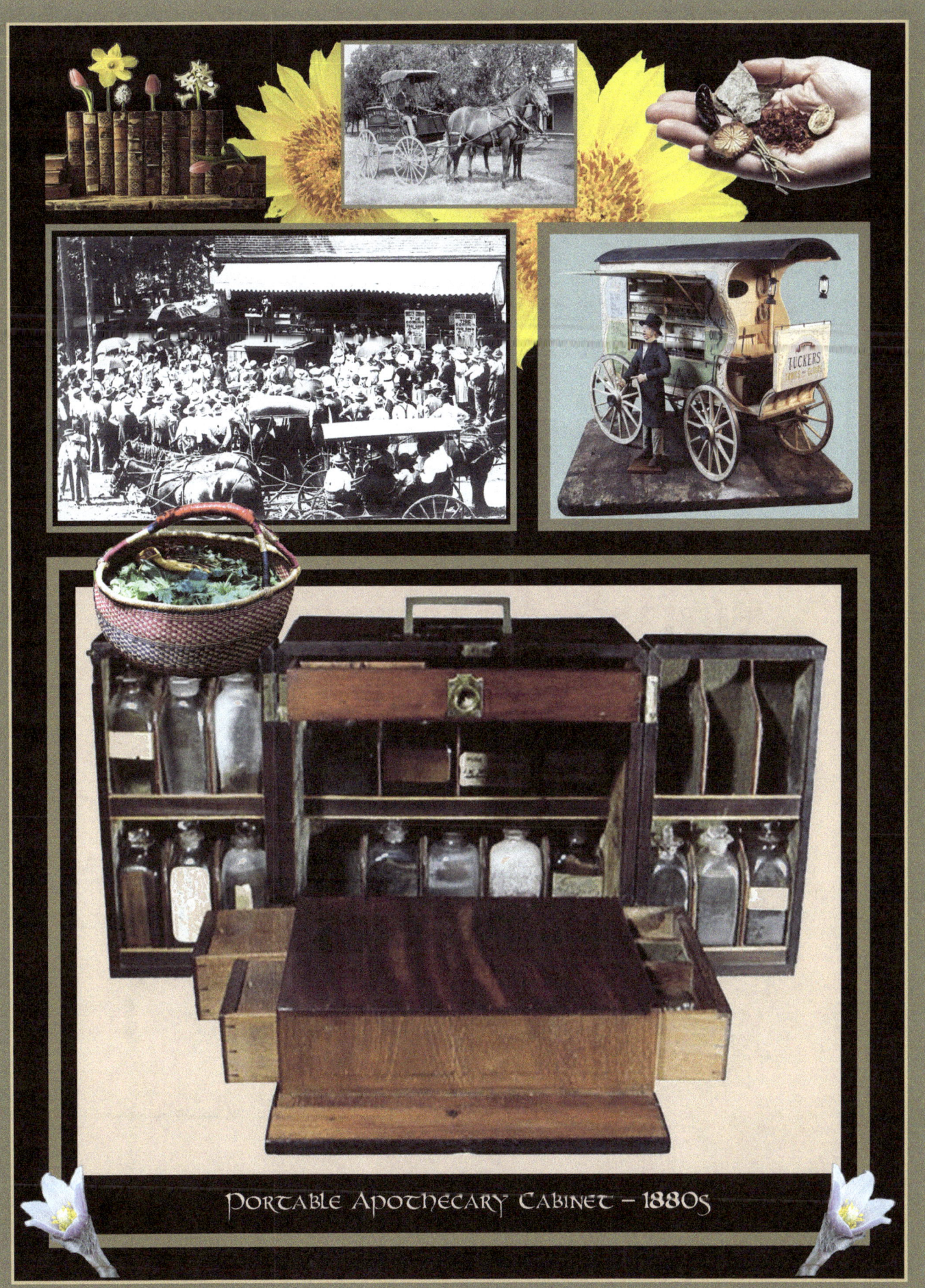

Portable Apothecary Cabinet – 1880s

By the early part of the 20th Century, the Medicine Wagon had evolved into hand-built trailers, the horsepower pulling them down the endless highway provided by trucks and automobiles.
Yet, nothing can strip them of those traits which define them most:
Their utter charm and undeniable enchantment.  Their service as a bridge between the healthful natural world and not always so healthy humankind.  Their wonderfully wandering ways.
And their furtherance of holistic healing whether or not it was permitted,
the purpose to which all Medicine Wagons are committed!

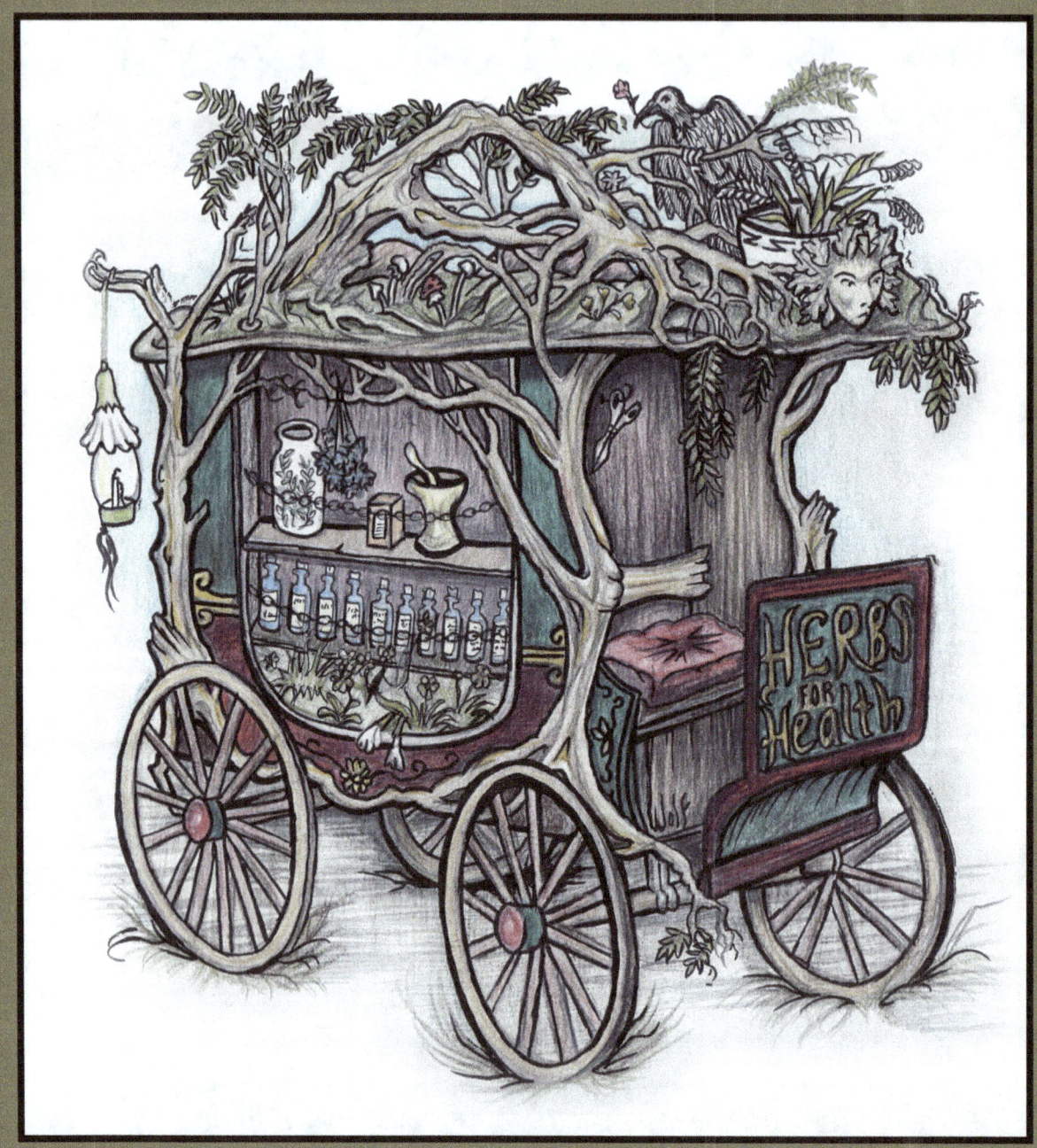

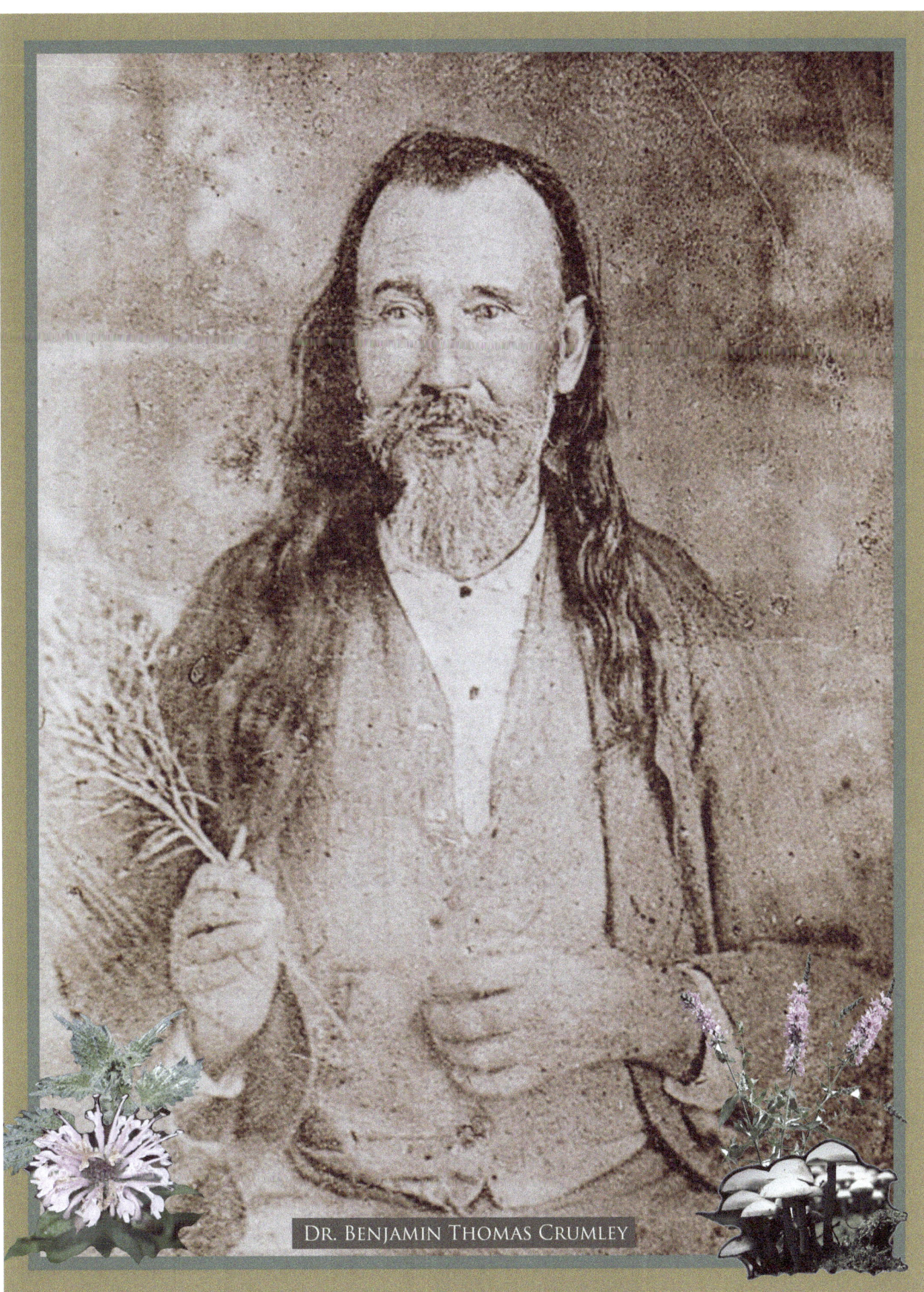
Dr. Benjamin Thomas Crumley

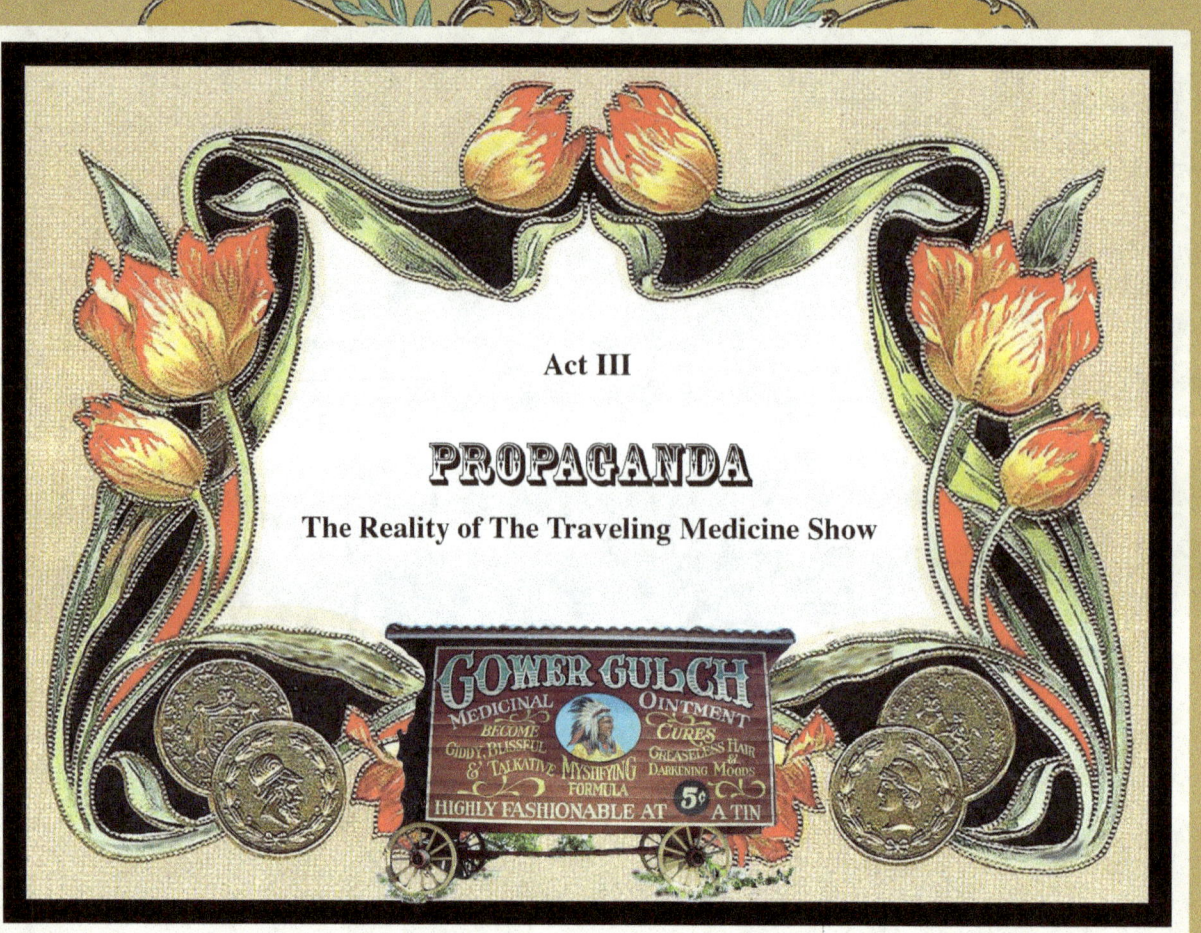

# Act III

# PROPAGANDA

## The Reality of The Traveling Medicine Show

All too often, the historic Medicine Shows are either demonized as dangerous money-grubbing scams, or else made fun of as quaint pieces of historic Americana. In the former case, there are those who consider all folk medicine not only inferior but treacherous, sounding as if anyone would have to be crazy to consider self medicating with plants, and as if licensed doctors and official experts were the infallible arbiters of what's good for us. In the latter, snide commentators herald the sensible benefits of modern medicine while showcasing herbalists and other natural healers as curious throwbacks, foolish children, superstitious primitives, naive practitioners of thankfully superseded healing practices.

Even many otherwise savvy people sometimes fall into the trap of accepting the anti-Medicine Show propaganda, accepting that our government was interested only in the health and protection of the paying public when they went after the medicine sellers with such a passion, while in reality it marked only the first of a long succession of legislative attacks against home remedies of all kinds, and herbalism in particular. These attacks were generated as a result of an organized campaign by the fast growing pharmaceutical industry and medical licensing agencies to ensure their monopolies on medicines and services, and thereby their ever more enormous profit margins. It was they who purchased the many thousands of dollars worth of ads branding all herbal concoctions as fraudulent and harmful "patent medicines," painting small manufacturers as the "grim reaper" in posters meant to scare housewives away from their neighborhood apothecaries, familiar poultices and teas and into pharmacies where they can purchase supposedly safe and miraculous drugs.

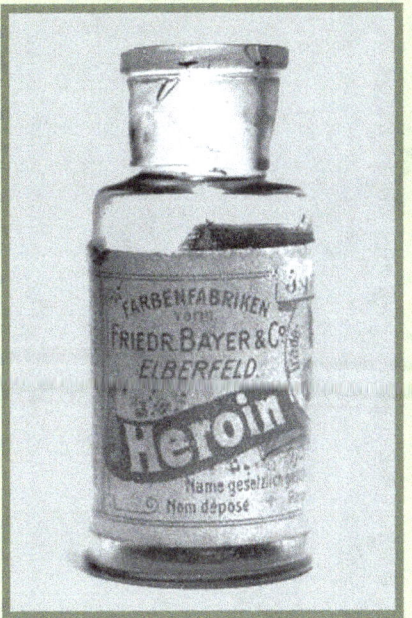

Between 1890 and 1910, before being labled by the government as "bad", baby-aspirin maker Bayer pushed processed heroin, with researchers touting it as a "nonaddictive" replacement for opium, while cocaine was being billed as an "instantaneous cure" for toothache. Relief it afforded, but a cure it wasn't.

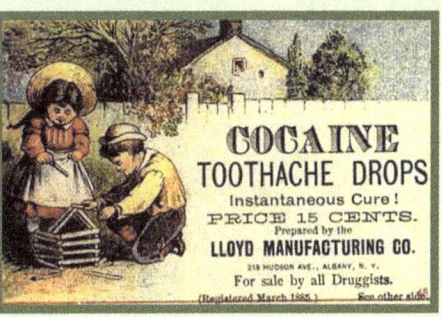

Metcalf's, Maltine and Mariani were just 2 of the hundreds of cocaine wines popular in America at one time. Pope Leo XIII awarded the maker Mariani a Vatican gold medal, and is said to have carried a bottle with him at all times.

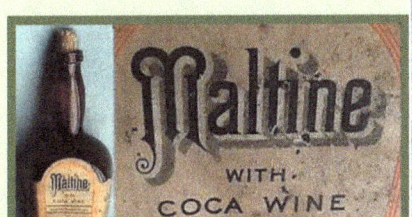

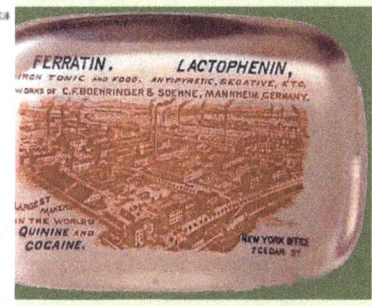

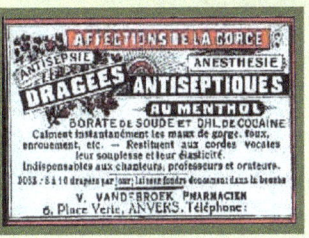

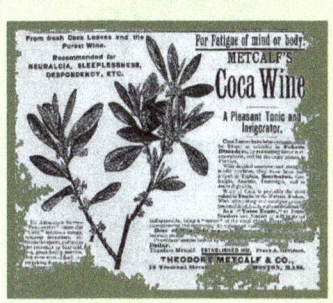

This historic collage should serve as a reminder not only that the administering of isolated or synthesized compounds is generally more dangerous and less healthful than using whole plants, or that greedy pharmaceutical companies can be indifferent to the suffering and addiction they so often contribute to... but that what we are being told is good for us by "experts", scientists and agency heads changes constantly. The lesson here is that it's unwise to trust the proclamations of so called authorities, that it can be highly unreasonable for us to heed their ever shifting recommendations or march in step to their every regulation. What the image of federally approved, opium-laced baby tonic should indicate, is the degree to which we need to trust our personal studies, intuition and experiences, with the responsibility for the well-being of ourselves and those we care about falling squarely on us. -Jesse Wolf Hardin

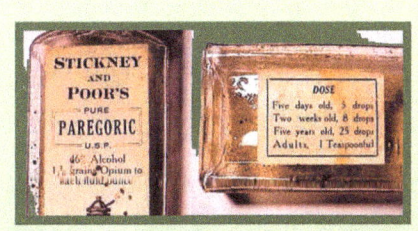

Critics then and now, point out that the main ingredient of herbal and vegetable nostrums was alcohol, and that their popularity depended on the drunken effects and the quantity of sales to drinkers in legally "dry" counties of the United States. In truth, these nostrums averaged from 5 to 15% alcohol, only in a few cases more than was needed to extract and preserve a medicinal tincture. Someone would have to be very thirsty for a buzz to drink the up to 10 bottles that would be required to experience a high, and the cost would be considerably more than simply buying a flask of bootlegged moonshine.

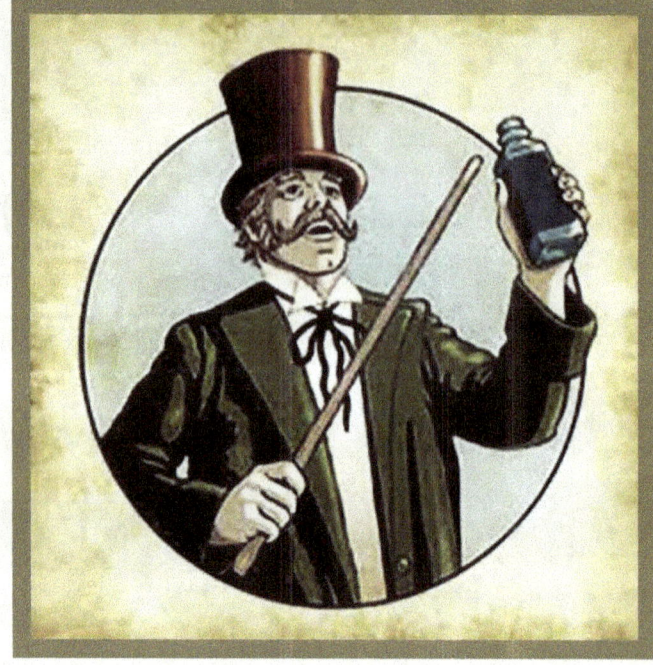

As the poster on the previous page shows, both opium and cocaine could be found in potions meant for pain, and scarily in recipes sold to "quiet the crying of babies, make them immune to the symptoms of colic, and guarantee a full nights sleep." Not only was heroin the primary active agent in the original Bayer pain pills, but also, cocaine the source of the "added energy" promised in Coca-Cola soda drink ads from the time of its inception.

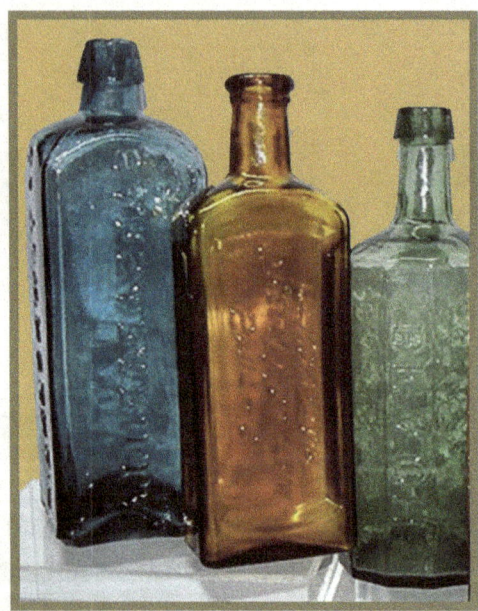

Some pitchmen sold watered down products, used "shills" in the audience to give false testimonials and encourage sales, or even ducked out of the area in the middle of the night in order to avoid complaints, refunds, or the strong arm of local law enforcement that could follow an exposition.

Their aim may have sometimes been no more than the income – the "velvet" that the shows produced – but far more often the mission and goals of the travelling medicine man was as much to make people feel better as it was to make money. Sellers often manufactured their own medicines, using folk recipes they researched on their own, or recipes commonly found in the popular manuals of their time such as 1882's "The Complete Herbalist," and the "King's American Dispensatory" published in 1898. The traveling show was often the only medical education or assistance that a community's residents ever received, and mobile doctors and "circuit dentists" could be not only a source of relief but a veritable lifesaver.

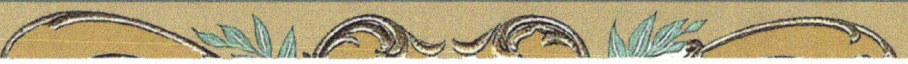

The European settlers brought to the world a long and respected tradition of medical herbalism, as well as bringing with them seeds for growing many of their favorite species from the "old world" to the new. That tradition was bolstered and amended by an infusion of herbal wisdom by the indigenous peoples of the Americas, with "Indian potions" proving far more helpful and far less destructive than the more "civilized" medical practices of the 18th Century. Those colonists who were financially well off could (unfortunately, as it were) afford the most "scientific" of treatments such as purging and blistering. First U.S. President George Washington might have survived to old age if not killed by the professional doctors who insisted on treating his condition by bleeding him, and the must esteemed modernist Dr. Benjamin Rush promoted dreadful doses of poisonous Calomel in many of the "improved" medicinal preparations well-to-do folks paid so much silver for.

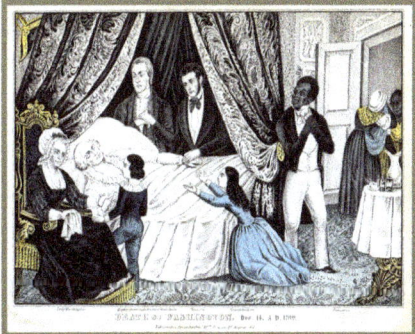

Fortunately for the "common man," the average working couple, they were mostly impoverished enough to still look to the fields, mountains and gardens for botanical relief for what ailed them, and otherwise to barter for the help of local herb-wise midwives. Out in "the country," when on occasion a local sheriff arrested the members of a traveling Medicine Show or forced them to move on, it seldom had anything to do with the quality or contents of the medicine being sold, but far more often was a response to what they considered to be the "lewd and immoral" nature of the show's dance routines!

Homemade herbal preparations sometimes became known as "recipes" or "receipts" to those who used them, but were falsely referred to as "patent medicines" by the professionals and competing manufacturers who sought their restriction. In actuality, there were no patent medicines in the new country. Patent medicines were the patented and licensed products of Great Britain, resented by Americans for their high cost and debatable qualities, and closest approximated in this country by the big government-licensed pharmaceutical corporations... who helped launch and largely funded what would become a campaign against herbalism – characterized as a defense of the people against "the patent medicine threat."

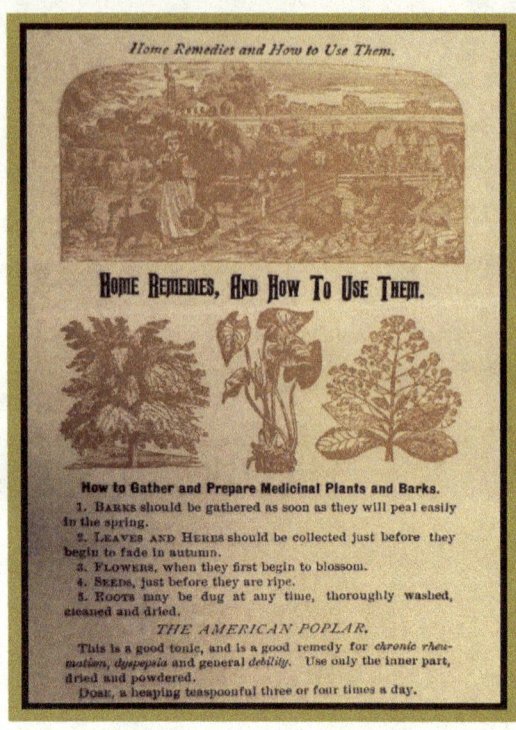

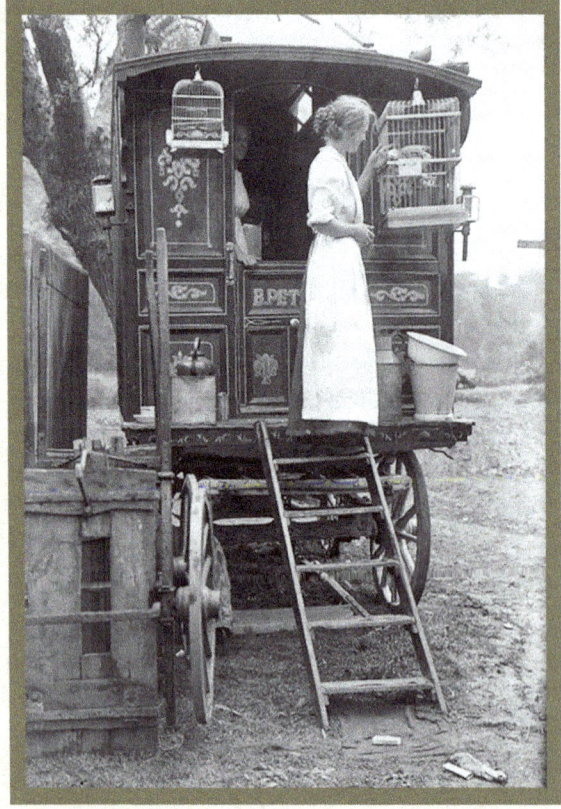

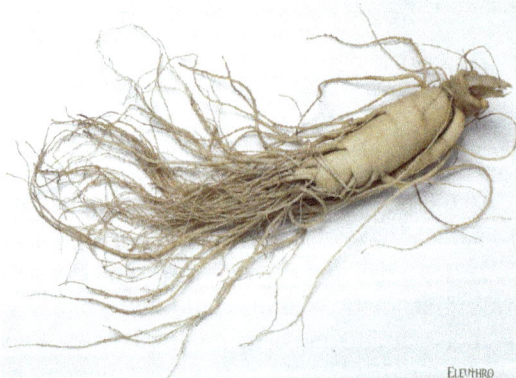

The threat that they really hoped to put a stop to, was the threat posed to their profitable paradigm by people learning how to take care of themselves and each other, using plant matter either homegrown or freely gathered.

And few did more to both spread and affirm the rebellious philosophies of self sufficiency and community health care than the traveling Medicine Shows we describe here.

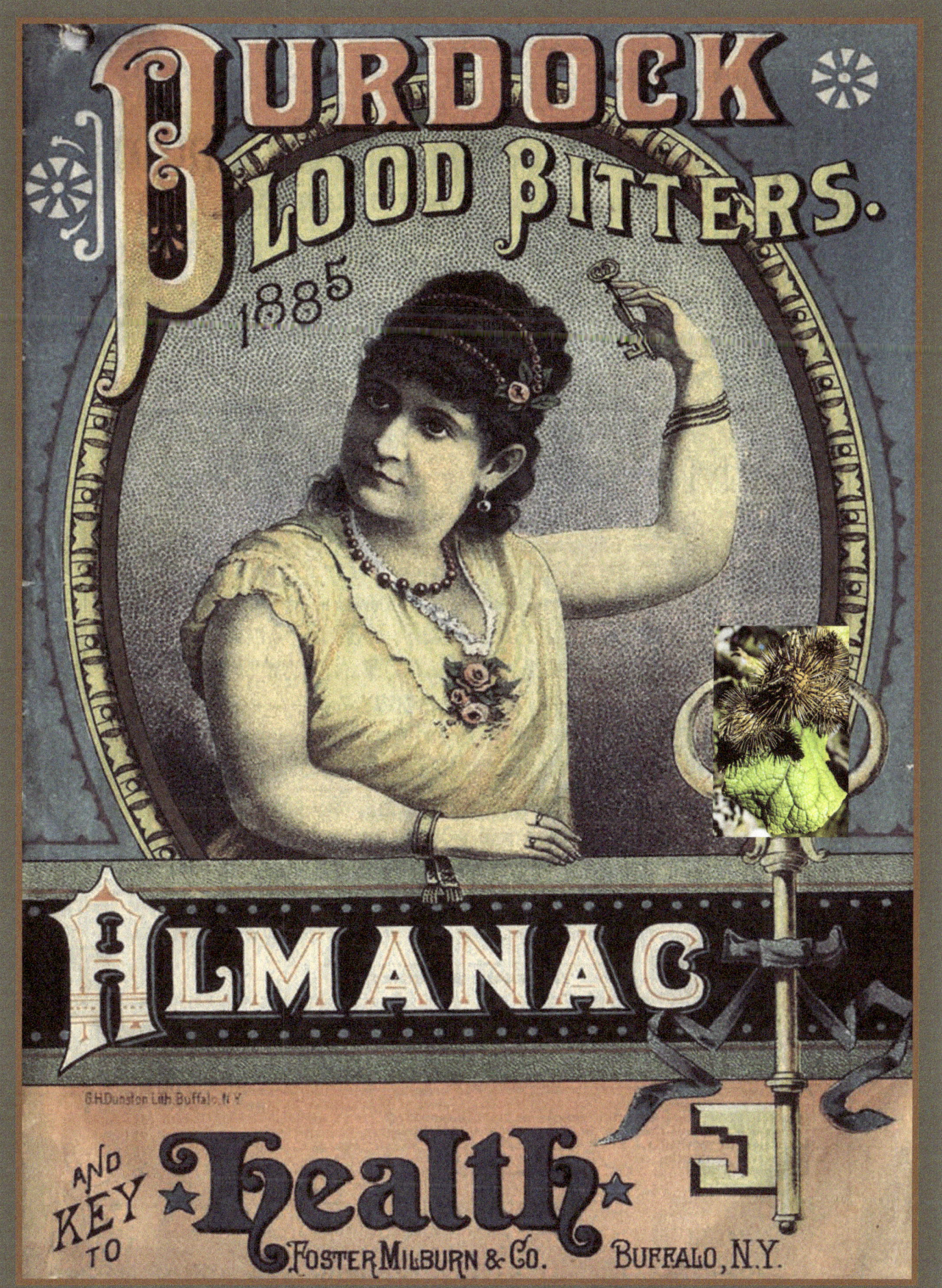

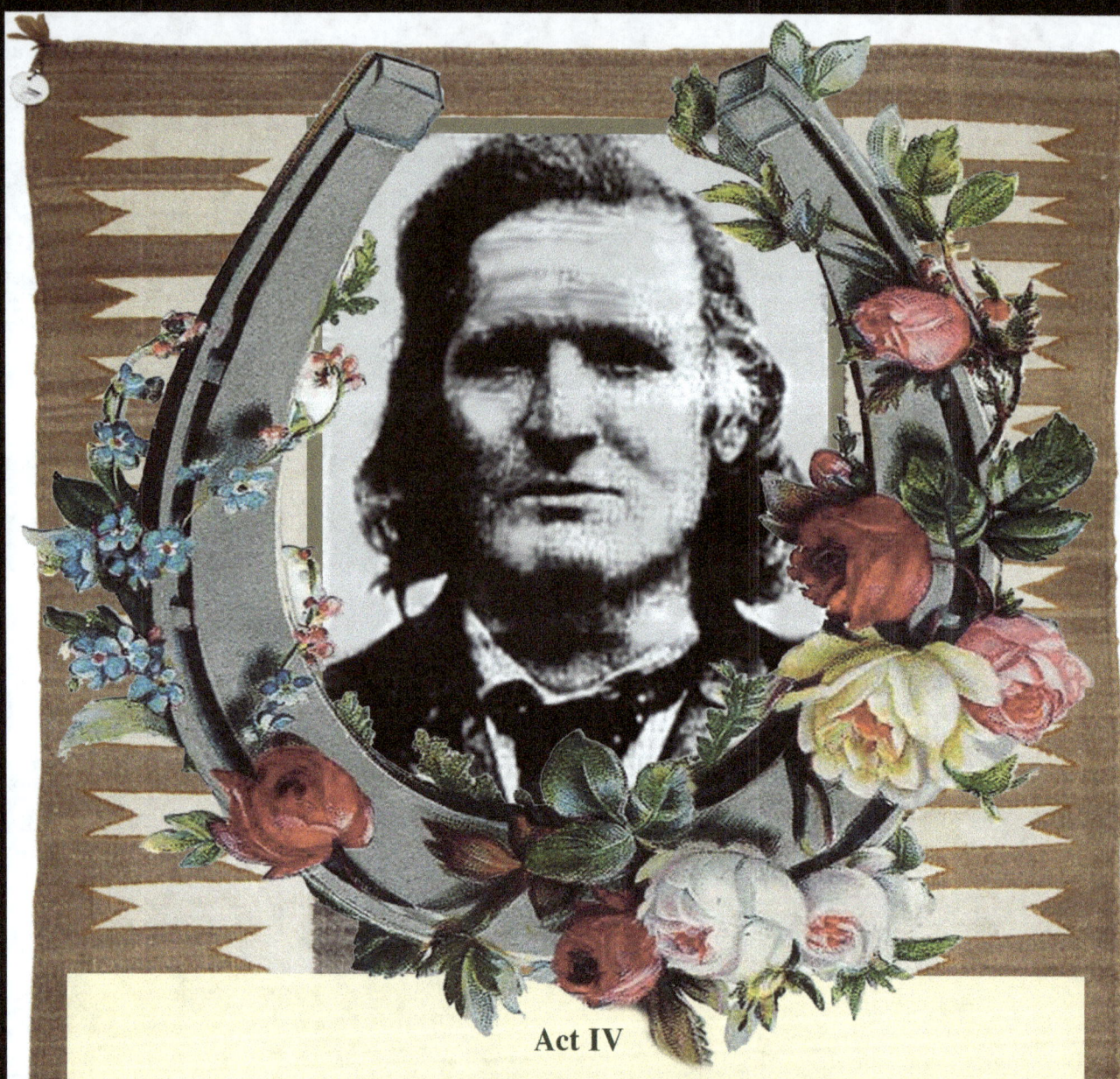

## Act IV

### JACOB "INDIAN JOHN" DERRINGER

*"I can not cure scarlet fever or diphtheria, but in some plant the father-of-all has provided a cure for these scourges. The fountain of health is all about, in backyards, fields, and along the watercourses."*
—Indian John Derringer

John Jacob Derringer was over six feet in height, with long ebony hair that rested on his shoulders, and usually wearing a black suit and hat to match. His well-used Medicine Wagon was a small buckboard affair featuring large copper tanks and pulled by a pair of black and white spotted Paint ponies, atop which he sat most erect and proud. His countenance was described by many of his 1880s Kansas Territory clients as "stoic" and even "grim," fixed as it was with the intensity of a true hell-and-brimstone preacher.

Native Americans have long been considered to be closer to nature, trusted with natural healing secrets unavailable to others. For this reason, it became de rigeur for large Medicine Shows to feature "Indians" along with "Orientals," and magicians in a night's performance. While there were many "white men" on the circuit posing as wizened chiefs in feathered headdresses to sell their products, "Indian John" Derringer most likely descended from mixed blood ancestry connecting him to the indigenous American healing tradition,

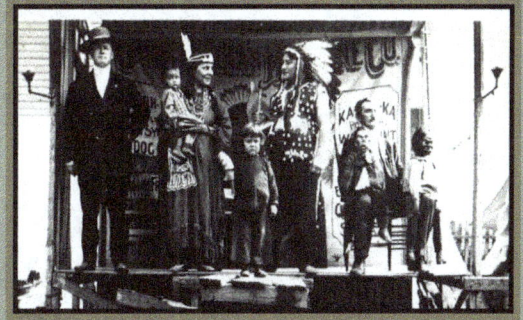

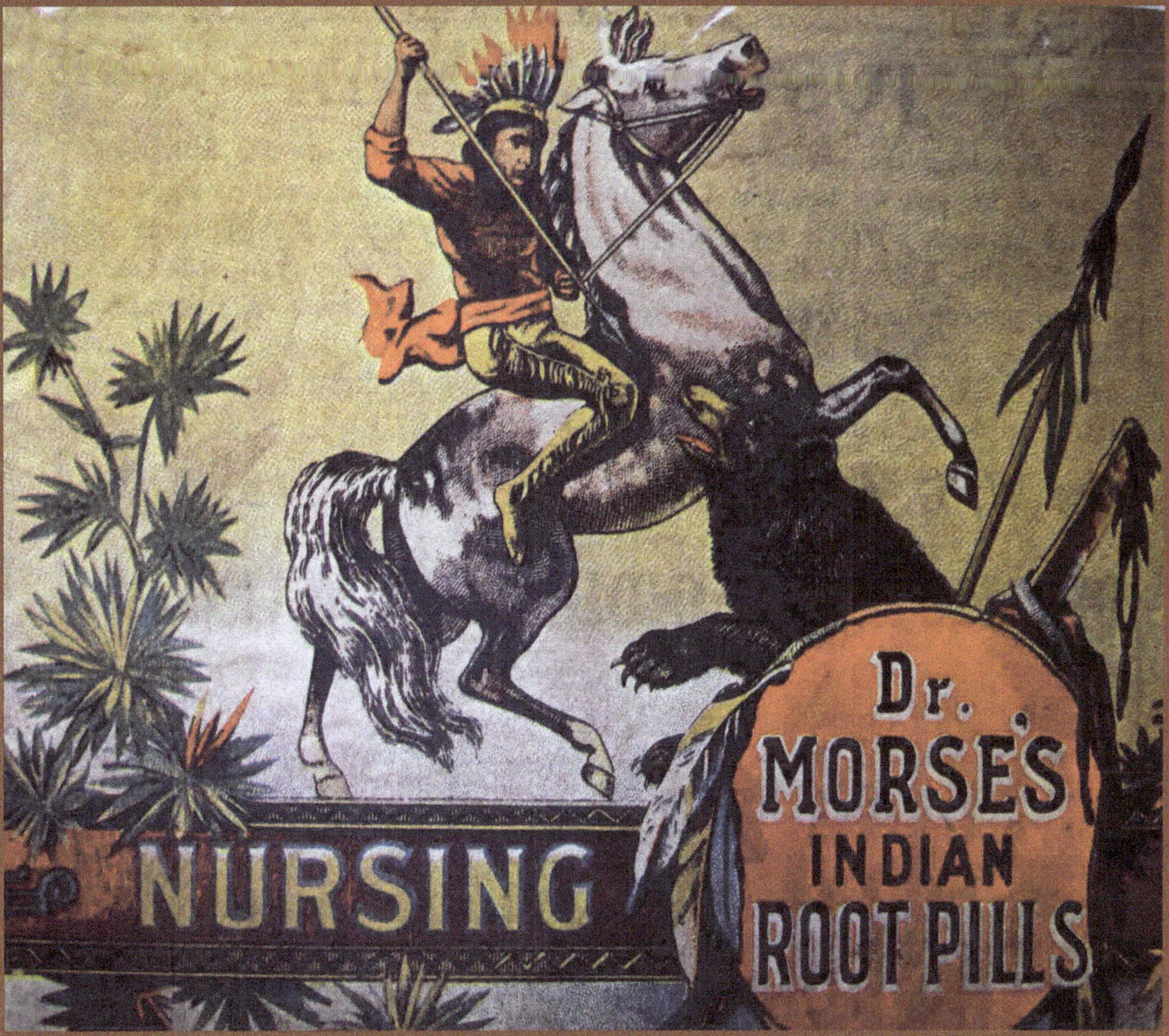

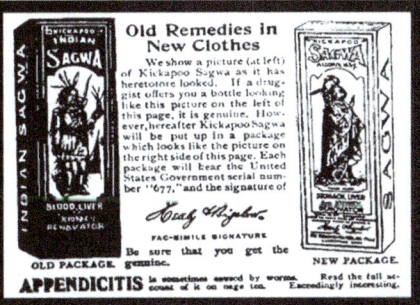

It was also exceedingly common for large commercial sellers to name their products "Indian" medicines, regardless of their source or attribution. Businesses like the far reaching Kickapoo company used dark skinned actors to do their marketing, growing into a big, dodgy company – creating the mold for the disreputable pharaceutical industries that followed. Some of these commercial "cures" were very helpful, just as are many modern drugs, but both were a step removed from the hands-on medicine making of herbalists like Jacob Derringer.

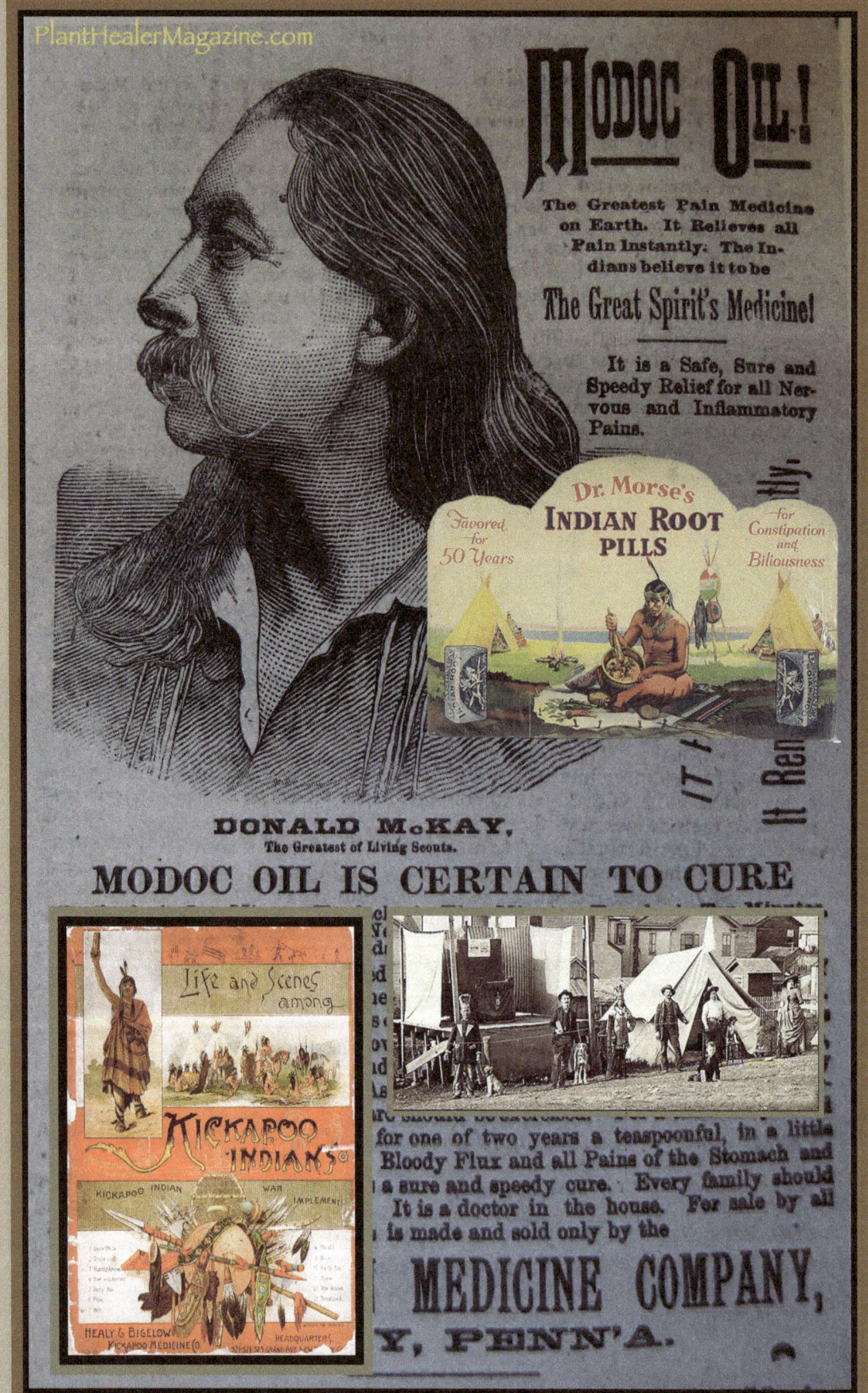

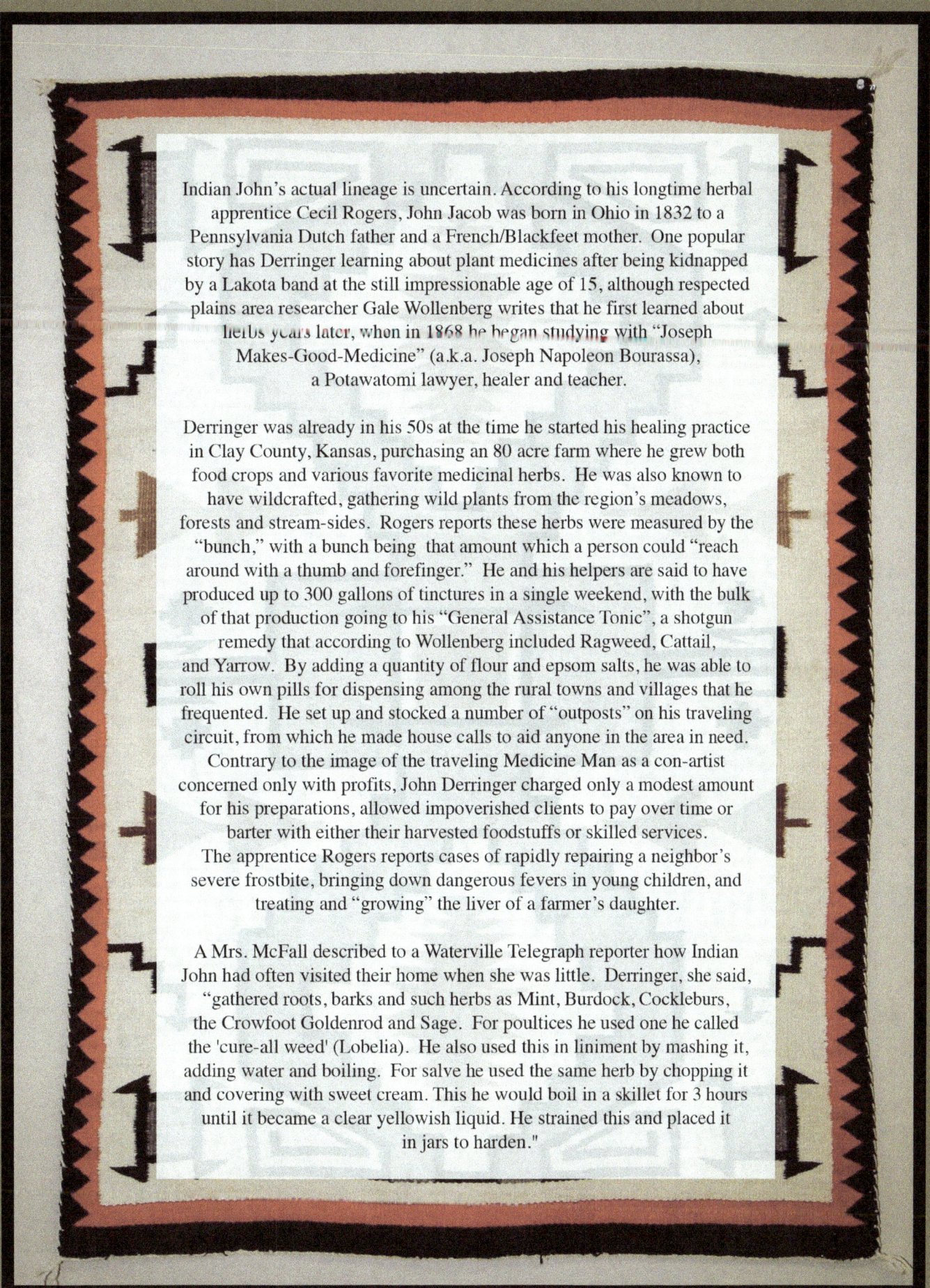

Indian John's actual lineage is uncertain. According to his longtime herbal apprentice Cecil Rogers, John Jacob was born in Ohio in 1832 to a Pennsylvania Dutch father and a French/Blackfeet mother. One popular story has Derringer learning about plant medicines after being kidnapped by a Lakota band at the still impressionable age of 15, although respected plains area researcher Gale Wollenberg writes that he first learned about herbs years later, when in 1868 he began studying with "Joseph Makes-Good-Medicine" (a.k.a. Joseph Napoleon Bourassa), a Potawatomi lawyer, healer and teacher.

Derringer was already in his 50s at the time he started his healing practice in Clay County, Kansas, purchasing an 80 acre farm where he grew both food crops and various favorite medicinal herbs. He was also known to have wildcrafted, gathering wild plants from the region's meadows, forests and stream-sides. Rogers reports these herbs were measured by the "bunch," with a bunch being that amount which a person could "reach around with a thumb and forefinger." He and his helpers are said to have produced up to 300 gallons of tinctures in a single weekend, with the bulk of that production going to his "General Assistance Tonic", a shotgun remedy that according to Wollenberg included Ragweed, Cattail, and Yarrow. By adding a quantity of flour and epsom salts, he was able to roll his own pills for dispensing among the rural towns and villages that he frequented. He set up and stocked a number of "outposts" on his traveling circuit, from which he made house calls to aid anyone in the area in need.

Contrary to the image of the traveling Medicine Man as a con-artist concerned only with profits, John Derringer charged only a modest amount for his preparations, allowed impoverished clients to pay over time or barter with either their harvested foodstuffs or skilled services.

The apprentice Rogers reports cases of rapidly repairing a neighbor's severe frostbite, bringing down dangerous fevers in young children, and treating and "growing" the liver of a farmer's daughter.

A Mrs. McFall described to a Waterville Telegraph reporter how Indian John had often visited their home when she was little. Derringer, she said, "gathered roots, barks and such herbs as Mint, Burdock, Cockleburs, the Crowfoot Goldenrod and Sage. For poultices he used one he called the 'cure-all weed' (Lobelia). He also used this in liniment by mashing it, adding water and boiling. For salve he used the same herb by chopping it and covering with sweet cream. This he would boil in a skillet for 3 hours until it became a clear yellowish liquid. He strained this and placed it in jars to harden."

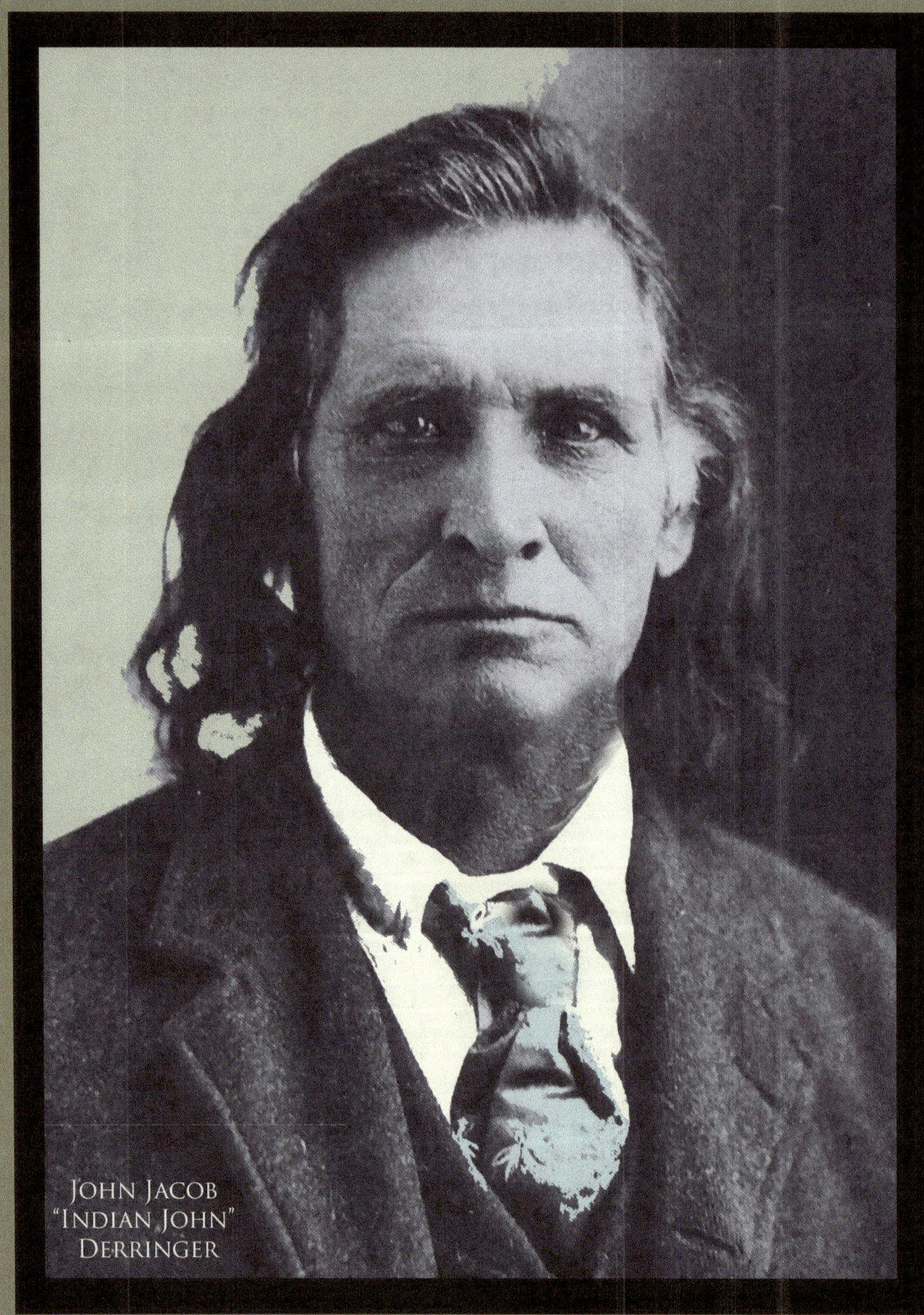

John Jacob "Indian John" Derringer

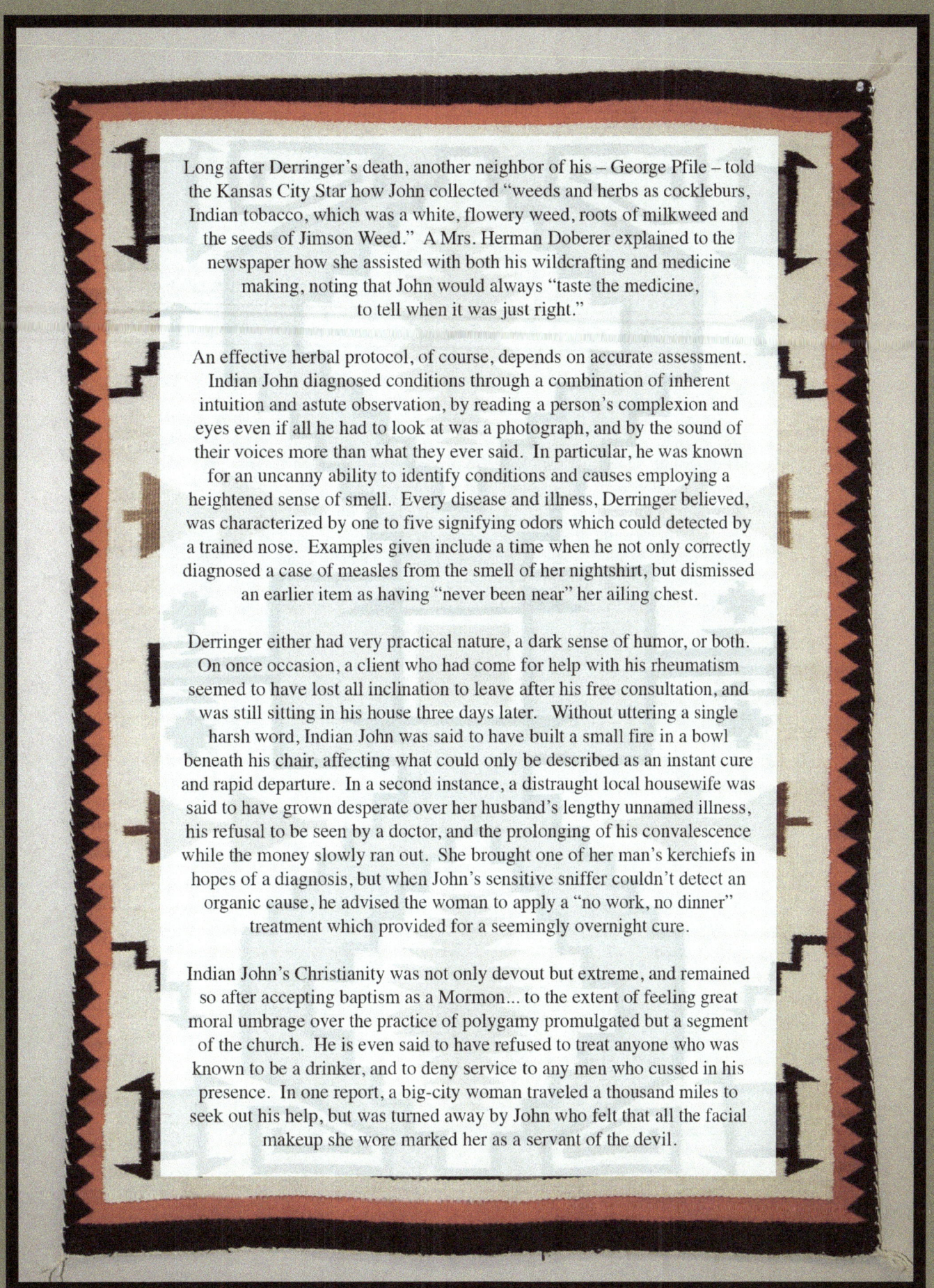

Long after Derringer's death, another neighbor of his – George Pfile – told the Kansas City Star how John collected "weeds and herbs as cockleburs, Indian tobacco, which was a white, flowery weed, roots of milkweed and the seeds of Jimson Weed." A Mrs. Herman Doberer explained to the newspaper how she assisted with both his wildcrafting and medicine making, noting that John would always "taste the medicine, to tell when it was just right."

An effective herbal protocol, of course, depends on accurate assessment. Indian John diagnosed conditions through a combination of inherent intuition and astute observation, by reading a person's complexion and eyes even if all he had to look at was a photograph, and by the sound of their voices more than what they ever said. In particular, he was known for an uncanny ability to identify conditions and causes employing a heightened sense of smell. Every disease and illness, Derringer believed, was characterized by one to five signifying odors which could detected by a trained nose. Examples given include a time when he not only correctly diagnosed a case of measles from the smell of her nightshirt, but dismissed an earlier item as having "never been near" her ailing chest.

Derringer either had very practical nature, a dark sense of humor, or both. On once occasion, a client who had come for help with his rheumatism seemed to have lost all inclination to leave after his free consultation, and was still sitting in his house three days later. Without uttering a single harsh word, Indian John was said to have built a small fire in a bowl beneath his chair, affecting what could only be described as an instant cure and rapid departure. In a second instance, a distraught local housewife was said to have grown desperate over her husband's lengthy unnamed illness, his refusal to be seen by a doctor, and the prolonging of his convalescence while the money slowly ran out. She brought one of her man's kerchiefs in hopes of a diagnosis, but when John's sensitive sniffer couldn't detect an organic cause, he advised the woman to apply a "no work, no dinner" treatment which provided for a seemingly overnight cure.

Indian John's Christianity was not only devout but extreme, and remained so after accepting baptism as a Mormon... to the extent of feeling great moral umbrage over the practice of polygamy promulgated but a segment of the church. He is even said to have refused to treat anyone who was known to be a drinker, and to deny service to any men who cussed in his presence. In one report, a big-city woman traveled a thousand miles to seek out his help, but was turned away by John who felt that all the facial makeup she wore marked her as a servant of the devil.

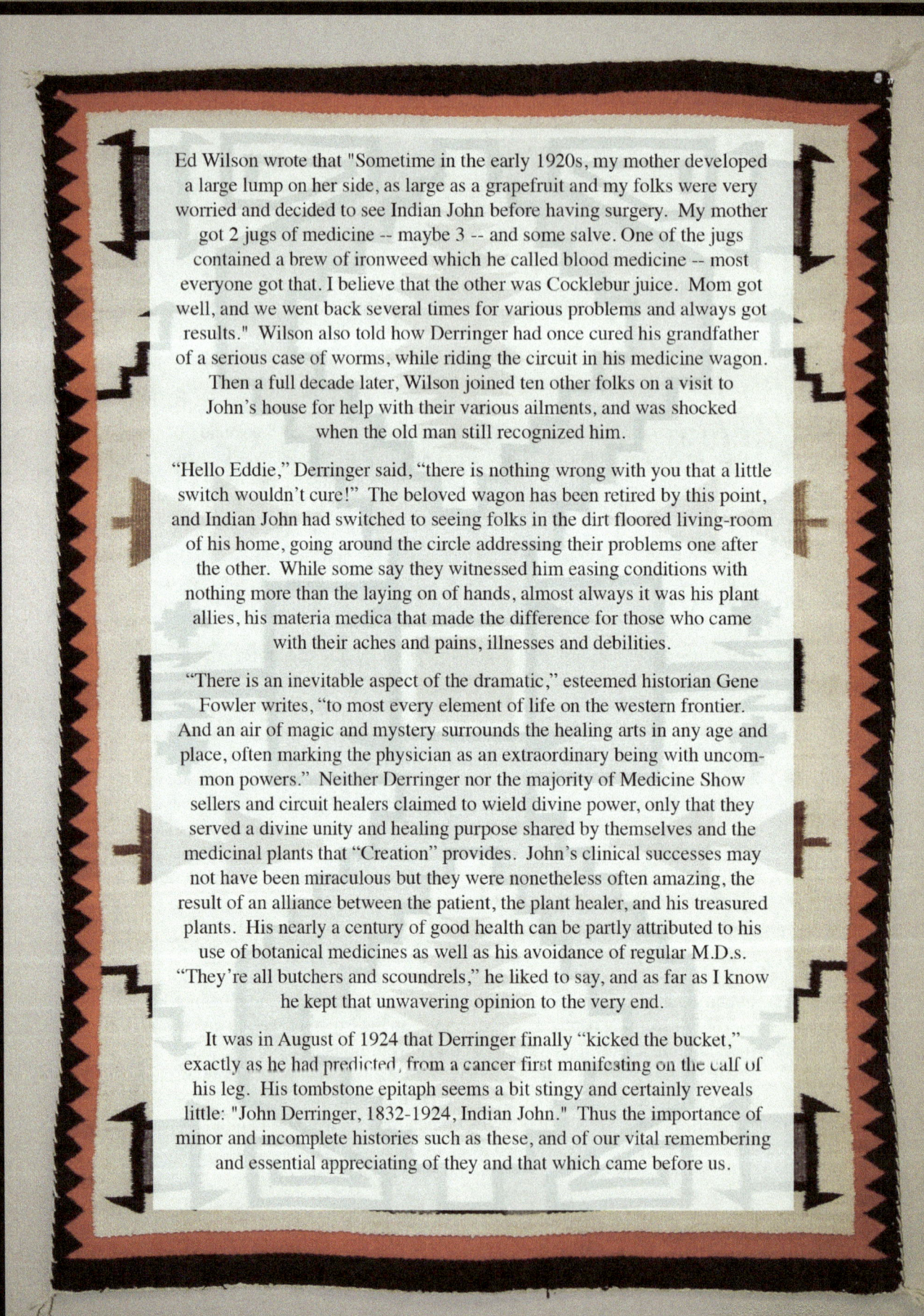

Ed Wilson wrote that "Sometime in the early 1920s, my mother developed a large lump on her side, as large as a grapefruit and my folks were very worried and decided to see Indian John before having surgery. My mother got 2 jugs of medicine -- maybe 3 -- and some salve. One of the jugs contained a brew of ironweed which he called blood medicine -- most everyone got that. I believe that the other was Cocklebur juice. Mom got well, and we went back several times for various problems and always got results." Wilson also told how Derringer had once cured his grandfather of a serious case of worms, while riding the circuit in his medicine wagon. Then a full decade later, Wilson joined ten other folks on a visit to John's house for help with their various ailments, and was shocked when the old man still recognized him.

"Hello Eddie," Derringer said, "there is nothing wrong with you that a little switch wouldn't cure!" The beloved wagon has been retired by this point, and Indian John had switched to seeing folks in the dirt floored living-room of his home, going around the circle addressing their problems one after the other. While some say they witnessed him easing conditions with nothing more than the laying on of hands, almost always it was his plant allies, his materia medica that made the difference for those who came with their aches and pains, illnesses and debilities.

"There is an inevitable aspect of the dramatic," esteemed historian Gene Fowler writes, "to most every element of life on the western frontier. And an air of magic and mystery surrounds the healing arts in any age and place, often marking the physician as an extraordinary being with uncommon powers." Neither Derringer nor the majority of Medicine Show sellers and circuit healers claimed to wield divine power, only that they served a divine unity and healing purpose shared by themselves and the medicinal plants that "Creation" provides. John's clinical successes may not have been miraculous but they were nonetheless often amazing, the result of an alliance between the patient, the plant healer, and his treasured plants. His nearly a century of good health can be partly attributed to his use of botanical medicines as well as his avoidance of regular M.D.s. "They're all butchers and scoundrels," he liked to say, and as far as I know he kept that unwavering opinion to the very end.

It was in August of 1924 that Derringer finally "kicked the bucket," exactly as he had predicted, from a cancer first manifesting on the calf of his leg. His tombstone epitaph seems a bit stingy and certainly reveals little: "John Derringer, 1832-1924, Indian John." Thus the importance of minor and incomplete histories such as these, and of our vital remembering and essential appreciating of they and that which came before us.

Never one to smoke tobacco, Derringer was known to occasionally enjoy drawing on a burl pipe packed with his favorite herbs. I like to picture him driven by his caring purpose towards the homes and people that need him, riding sternly atop his bouncing and jarring buckboard, his medicines sloshing in their containers in the back, his eyes blazing with purpose and alert, his nose taking in and evaluating every passing scent. One hand holds the twin reins directing his Paint horse team. The other lifts a pipe to the old man's mouth, from which curls a trail of sweet Mullein smoke that we in our own time and place can follow.

## John Jacob Derringer Concoctions

(excerpted from Gale Wollenberg's "Indian John: Volume 2: A look at Uncle John's Medicine Chest" – intended for historic interest only)

Blood Medicine or Tonic:
2 parts Hoary or Blue Vervain
1 part White or Prairie Sage
1 part Missouri Goldenrod

To Treat Swollen Mucus Membranes:
1 part Cocklebur, burrs only
1 part Balsam
1 part Common Burdock, burrs only

Kidney & Liver Medicine:
1 part Cottonwood inner bark
1 part Lead plant
1 part Sumac berries or Fennel

General System Medicine:
1 part Cattail
1 part Ragweed
1 part Fever Weed (or mint)
1 part Yarrow
1 part Rosin Weed
1 part Button Weed

Ulcer Medicine:
1 part Cocklebur leaves
1 part Sunflower leaves
1 part Sumac roots
1 part Choke Cherry bark

**Indian John Dies.**
John Derringer, aged 92 years, better known as "Indian John," passed away at his home near Fact, yesterday, at five p. m.
His extensive practice in making medicines of herbs and his healing of the sick made him many true friends who were greatly shocked by his sudden death.
Funeral services will be held at the home tomorrow morning at 9:30 a. m. Interment will be made in Idylwild cemetery.

For all of the above recipes, Derringer boiled the ingredients with water at more than 200 degrees. A pint was boiled for about 10 minutes; a gallon was boiled 1 1/2 hours. A "bunch" (the amount of stems and leaves that the thumb and forefinger can surround) is added to a gallon of water. For a pint, a "handful" of plant material would be brewed.

### To make the blood medicine in pill form:

Slow boil 1 gallon down to 2/3 pint. Mix 2 tablespoons of epsom salts into liquid thoroughly. Put in 1/3 pint of flour and mix to a stiff batter. Put into a dish and allow to cool 15 minutes and then form this dough into pills the size of a corn kernel. Dry in the sun until hard.

In Derringer's later years, he used a 3/8-inch hail screen over a wooden frame, rolled the dough out flat and pressed it through the screen to form little square pills. The pills were about 1/4-inch by 3/8-inch square.

### Medicinal Teas

Ragweed: Relieves hay fever/asthma applied to external swellings.
Mule Tail: Relieves arthritis, stops vomiting and diarrhea
Dandelion root: Relieves rheumatism
Choke Cherry bark and ragweed: Relieves hay fever
Dried Elderberry blossoms: Reduces fever
Evening Primrose Liniment
Fpr Poison Ivy rash, Poison Oak rash and sun allergy rash; relieves eczema

Take 1/2 gallon of Evening Primrose leaves, and pour over them 1 quart of boiling hot water. Let cool until you can work leaves with the hands. Knead and squeeze the leaves for 15 minutes, squeeze liquid off leaves and throw leaves away. The liquid is the liniment, ready for use. The curing time is from 3 to 5 minutes. Cure of the blistering stages of the rashes will take about 30 minutes.

### Poultices

For bad knees: Combine evening primrose liniment with mashed primrose leaves and extra water while slow boiling. Apply hot with cloth wrapping.

For burns: Remove thorns of prickly pear cactus and make leaves into a poultice. Apply daily.

For cancerous skin lesion: Crush leaves of evening primrose and apply to lesion. Leave on the lesion for 3 days.

To draw a boil to a head: Crush Hedge ball and make a poultice. Place on affected area for 4 hours every day, 2 hours on and 2 hours off and 2 hours on again.

For bedsores: Apply milkweed sap on sores.

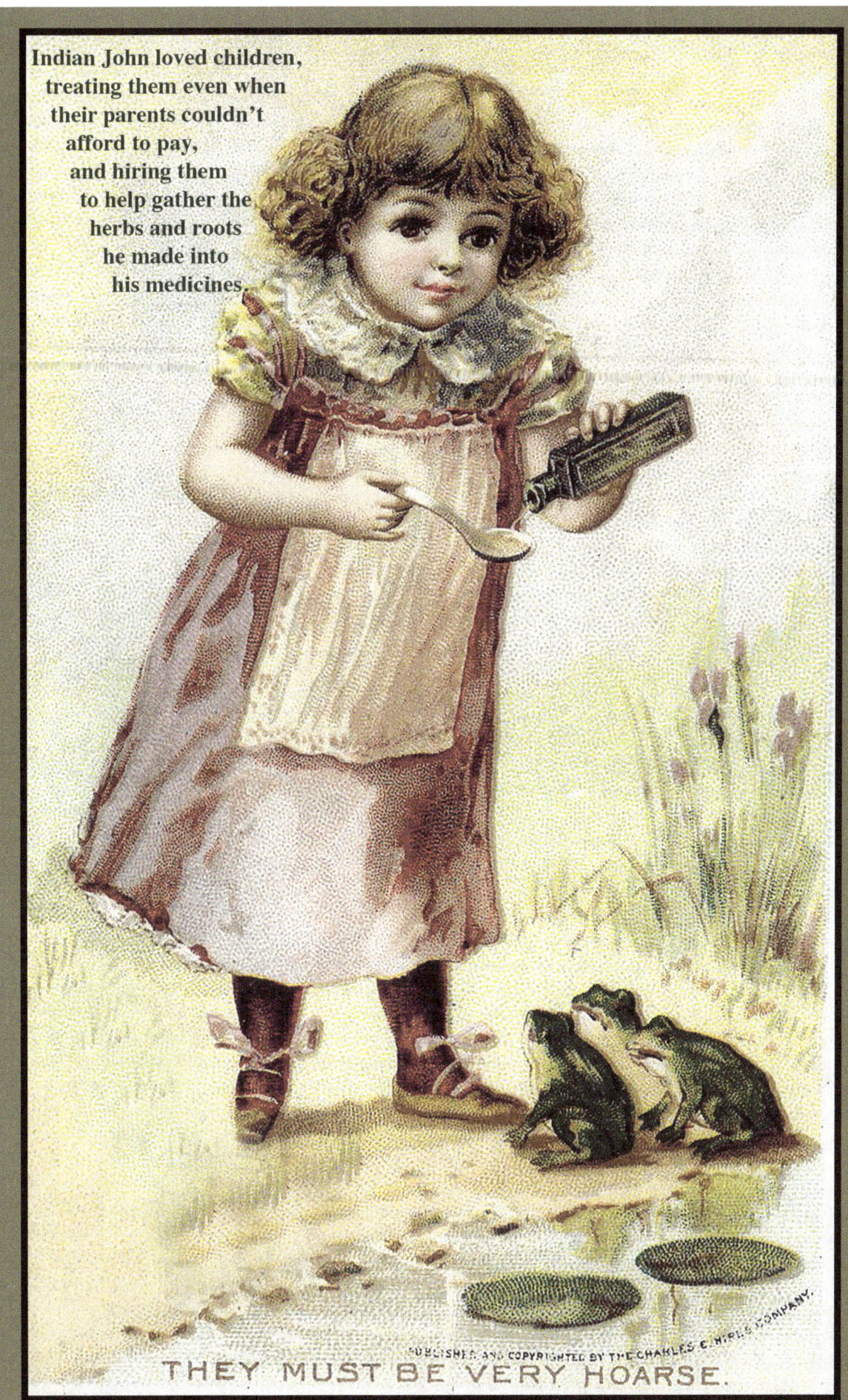

Act V

# J. I. LIGHTHALL

The "Diamond King"

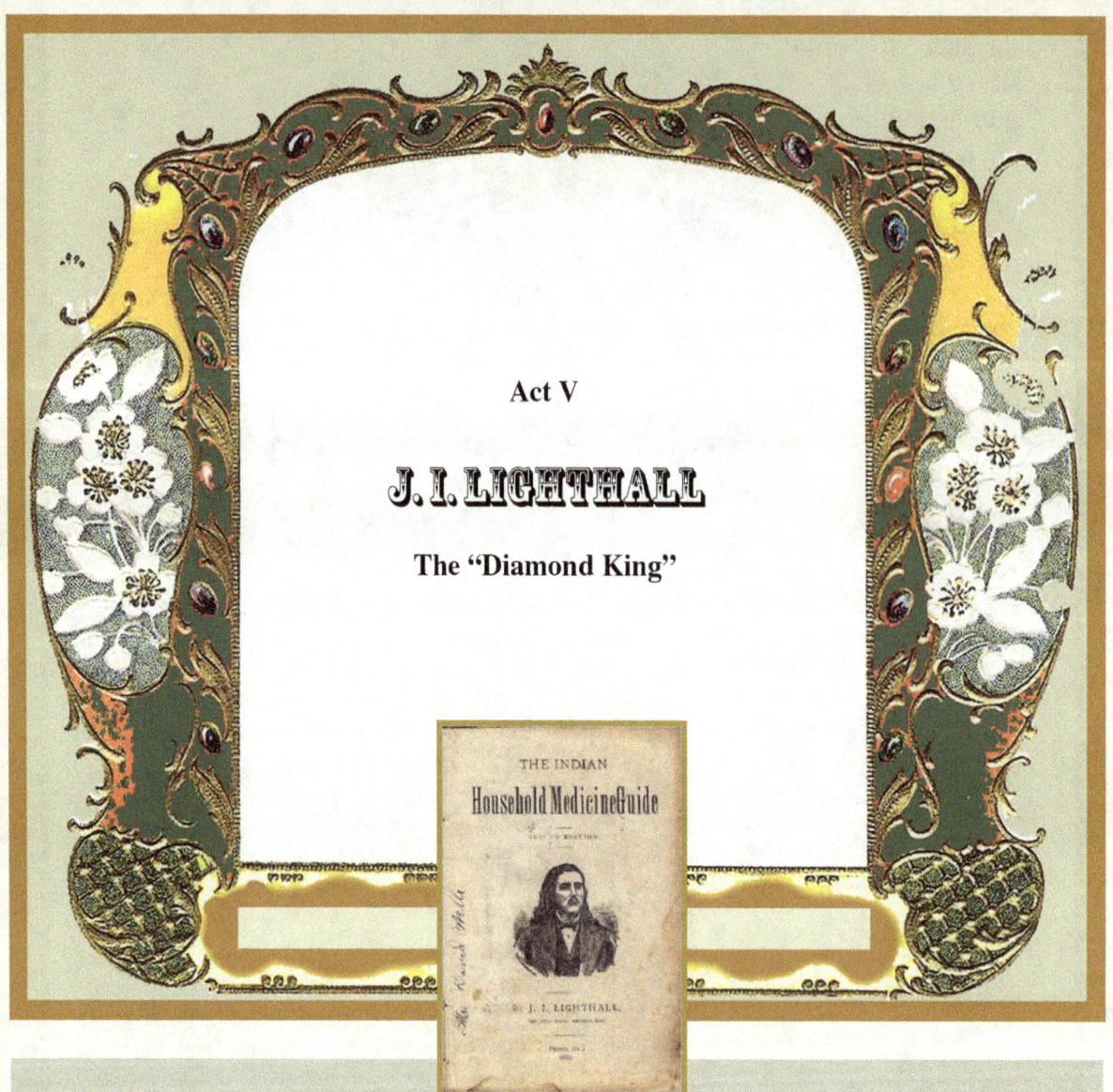

*"We are wonderfully made. We are a greater mystery to ourselves than all our surroundings."*
—J. I. Lighthall

Years later, folks liked to remember the first glimpses of the brightly painted wagons pulled by nobly dressed horses, growing slowly in size as they approached ever closer to the town limits. One held a handful of Indians in full regalia, a second carried a ventriloquist with a smiling "Mr. Healthy" dummy and wretched looking "Mr. Ill" propped on his knees, along with a band featuring trumpets and a giant bass drum. With each beat of drum, the man in the lead carriage tossed out another handful of nickels to the kids and adults now following eagerly behind, bending over to pick up the coins and then running to catch up. His great hat set back on the crown of his head, his long curly hair buoyed by the wind, the elaborately dressed gentleman was recognizable by all. Carefully placed articles in the newspaper would have long foretold of his coming, and advance riders had alerted the throngs that the show was soon to go on.

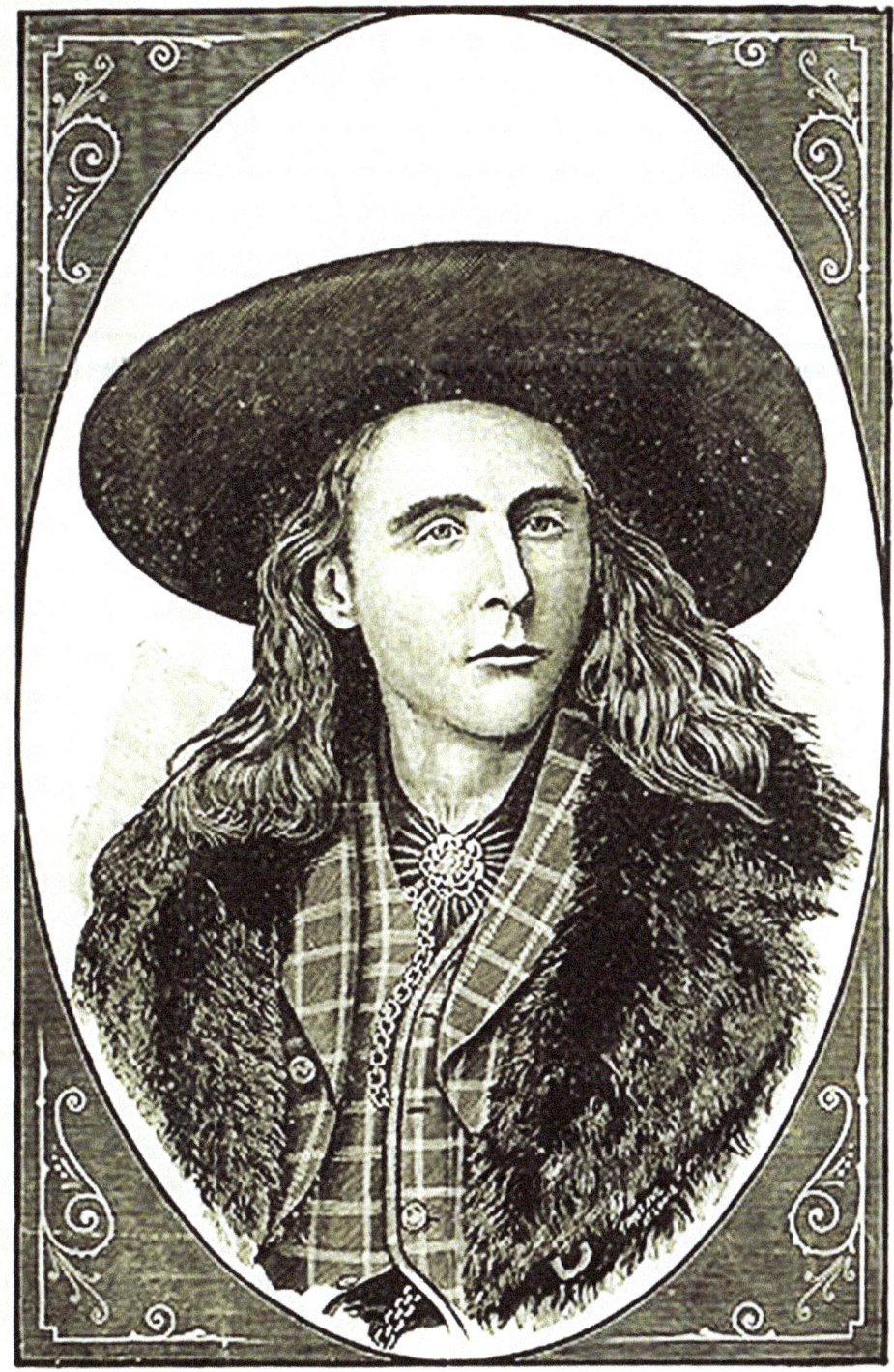

"The bills read: "Dr. Lighthall's most stupendous medicine show on Earth...
or in the other place."

J. I. Lighthall caused quite a stir in every Western town he visited with his wondrous Medicine Show, quickly becoming one of the most talked about characters of the American frontier. His name would regularly be mentioned in the same breath as other showmen like Wild Bill Hickock and Buffalo Bill Cody, though famed for his glorious hawking of herbal medicines rather than any feats of scouting or dusty-street shootouts. Often stories circulated about the efficiency and speed at which various gunfighters had silenced their opponents, with such dazzling figures as "killed three men with four shots," or "four people shot in less time than it takes to tell it"... while in contrast, James Lighthall's oft recounted claim to fame was "extracting 14 people's teeth in 19 seconds."

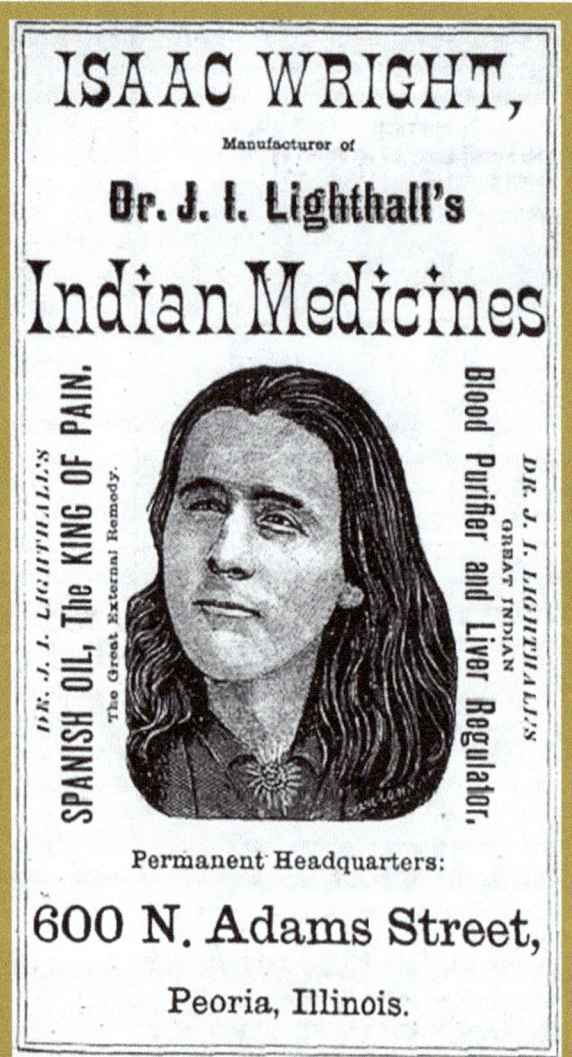

While there were many a Medicine Showman in the 1870s, none were splashier than these, and all in the business looked up to the man whose jewell encrusted vest and sombrero had caused him to be dubbed the "Diamond King." A typical Lighthall tent show would begin with musical selections, half of which were rousing patriotic songs with the rest being popular minstrel dance songs. A series of comedians, puppeteers and sometimes fire-eaters would be followed by the Diamond King offering free dental extractions to anyone in the audience.

In places where there were few dentists and few folks who could afford one, as much as a third of his audience might volunteer for the procedure. One witness reported the Doc "busy as a butcher preparing a barbecue for a firemen's picnic, hurling molars and incisors hight into the air like shooting stars on a dark night." The climax came when Lighthall himself stepped out onto the stage in a full length beaver fur coat with his dazzling crystal headed cane, and immediately launched into an impassioned spiel on the ailments of the time and the herbal nostrums brewed to treat them.

The following a small portion of Diamond King Lighthall's tract on medicine and Materia Medica. My partner Kiva Rose found that he downplayed the problems with using Senna regularly for the bowels, and that for some reason he shortchanged American Ginseng, calling it a "mild tonic fit for a boy." For the most part, however, he was pretty right on, and demonstrates a decent understanding of physiomedicalism.. Already, Doc Lighthall was aware of the tide against not only patent medicines but home preparations and granny doctors. The national Food and Drug Act of 1904 not only removed some dangerous or misleading products from the shelves of stores, it also spelled the first of many blows against folk medicine and herbalism.

Italics are added by this editor, to emphasize points and attitude most important to us today.

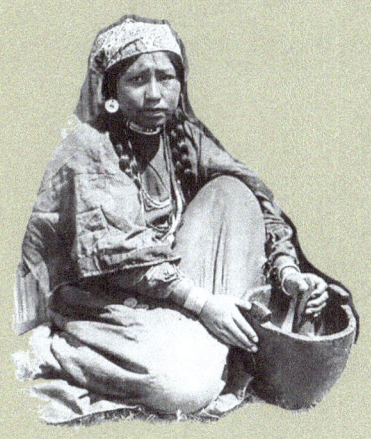

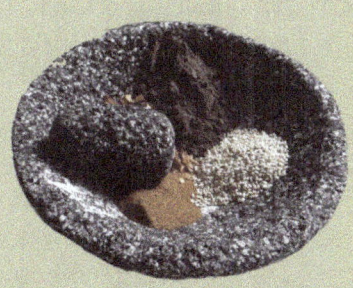

## The Indian Household Medicine Guide

by J. I. Lighthall (1883)

**To My Many Readers:**

...saying to you, use your own judgment, uninfluenced by any prejudice that may have previously existed in your minds. Give my advice a trial if you need it, and judge me and what I say by the effects. I give you my word and honor most solemnly, that all I have told you is safe for the most delicate person to try, without the slightest danger of producing any effect detrimental, either temporary or permanent. A wise person will glean knowledge from whatever source it may arise. The compass of the Indian is the moss on the north side of the tree, which is knowledge from a natural source gleaned by the wild untutored savage.

I will close by saying, good education is the only reliable means of lasting reforms, and that will teach people to think for themselves, and that simple medical facts have been hidden in the past by technical words, but to-day are told in common English.

*(From the Guidebook:)* Lighthall was born the 19th of January, in the year 1856, in Indiantown, or Tiskilwa, Bureau County, Illinois, where he received instructions, morally and educationally, until he arrived at the age of eleven years, when he left home with a youthful ambition to try his fortune in the west. He went to Kansas and the Indian Territory, where he formed a warm attachment for the Indians, and learned their ways and habits of life. It was a marked feature in his nature, from his infancy up, to be a close observer of Nature in reference to the vegetable kingdom. When but a boy he loved flowers, and wondered what kind of roots they had, and what they were good for; which indicated a natural gift for botany and the herbal kingdom, and when thrown among the Indians his mind was at once diverted by the Indian doctors, from the fact that they were all the time gathering roots, barks, leaves and flowers; consequently he would go with them into the mountains, hills, prairies, and woodlands, and assist them in gathering Nature's remedies and manufacturing them into Indian remedies. He at once observed the fact that the Indian doctors never injured their patients with their innocent remedies, and that they soon recovered without aching bones or a salivated mouth. From this fact he became strongly impressed with the fact that what was good for an Indian certainly was good for a white man, and that it was a duty he owed to civilization to introduce or bring before it the Indian Herbal Theory. The object of the author is to give each one the opportunity of learning how to care for his own system, and rectifying the wrongs that may assail it with harmless remedies, that will do good, and never harm when taken according to directions.

**A balm is hidden in the leaf,**
**That God has given for relief.**
**The Indians of the Western plains**
**Have found that they will cure our pains.**
**So now the author does extend**
**A helping hand, an honest friend.**
**He'll cure your aches, relieve your pain,**
**If you will buy his King of Pain.**
**It's made of barks, and oils, and leaves,**
**And seldom ever man deceives.**
**It never fails to satisfy,**
**And on it, friends, you can rely.**

### Medicine

Medicine, in its common acceptation in the minds of the people, is a substance that cures diseases, but the truth of the matter is, medicine never cured anything. It is the natural tendency of a majority of diseases to get well within themselves, free from medical aid. Medicine, properly administered, simply assists nature to remove the cause that obstructs her acting in a normal condition. Medicine is not a humbug. The humbug is in its improper administration. When medicine is properly administered it comes to the sufferer as a gift from God. Medicine is unjustly judged. It is not medicine that is at fault, but it is those who give it without the proper knowledge of its effects, and when it is indicated. Medicine, when it is not properly given, proves an actual poison to the system. The Indian Materia Medica treats of herbs and vegetation in general. That is, that part of vegetation which is known by them to have medicinal properties. They will never injure the system when conformed to according to directions given.

## Electicism -- The Free Thinker of Medicine

The right to choose the best from all of the one idea theories of medicine; liberty uncircumscribed by the teachings of fanatics; freedom to judge for yourself that which is best of all; that you can learn of the many ideas of medical men of the world. Love for all, hatred toward none; freedom of thought; the right to counsel with all, ungoverned by a mean disgraceful code of ethics. Liberty to exercise good common sense, and use that which is best calculated to do good in the case in which it is indicated. This is the true definition of Electicism. They are the most prosperous class of doctors on the face of the world, because they believe in personal liberty as well as general liberty, and that which is right, and hate smart fanatics.

## Quackopaths

There is a class of doctors that are drawn from all the schools of medicine that profess to be that which they are not. They may possess diplomas, but they got them upon examination day, by some student, that had studied hard and well and was naturally sharp, helping them and cheating the professors. They never merited a diploma. They spent their time in bar rooms and at billiard tables when they should have been burning midnight oil over Gray's Anatomy, or Huxley and Dalton's Physiology, in order that they might not butcher poor suffering humanity, and have more knowledge of the human system, and know better how to prescribe medicine to those who need it, and therefore this being a fact, every one should be on their guard. It is not the man that has the diploma that is always the good doctor. I know several men that have no diplomas, that are naturally inclined in that direction, that have good success, and are men that study the human organization and the effects of medicine on it, and try to improve their moments, in order that they may properly fit themselves for usefulness, and to benefit humanity. From the fact that so many force themselves through college, a diploma does not always signify that they are fit to prescribe or issue medicine. It is the man that makes medicine a study, and studies it constantly and diligently, thinking for himself, reasoning from cause to effect, using common sense in all things, and when he or they give medicine, are sure they are right, and give it so it won't do any harm if it does no good. There are more quacks that have diplomas than there are quacks that have not. I once knew a doctor that thought himself wise, and boasted over twenty-five years experience, and when I asked him about golden seal and black cohosh, he laughed at me, and said he had never stooped so low; that they were simply granny remedies. God pity such men.

## Marrubium Vulgare - Hoarhound

This is a harmless and yet a very important and useful remedy. It is found growing along creeks and rocky places, and should be gathered in the months of July and August.

Medical properties and uses. -- In order to get the full medical force of this plant a tea should be made from the green leaf and tops. It is especially an expectorant and diaphoretic. In this form I know of no remedy that will break up a cold on the lungs and bronchial tubes quicker than hot tea made from the hoarhound plant. It readily restores the arrested secretions to their normal standard. The way it should be used for colds on the lungs is as follows: Make a strong tea of the leaves and tops, sweeten with loaf sugar or honey, and take a hot foot bath, then drink the hot tea and immediately go to bed and cover up warm, and the result will be, in a majority of cases, free expectoration in twelve hours from the time it is taken.

## Inula Helenium - Elecampane

Elecampane is one of our many harmless, mild tonics. The root is the medical part of the plant, and by many highly appreciated. It is mild and slow in its effects, consequently should be continued a long time in order to accomplish the object for which it is taken.

Medical properties and uses. -- Elecampane is a mild tonic to the mucous linings and to the skin. It has been found by the Indian doctors to be of benefit in many skin diseases. It has a special affinity for the bronchial tubes and lungs in general. It is indicated where there is pain in the breast with considerable expectoration. It is better used with other remedies of similar proprieties.
I will now give you an Indian formula:
Elecampane Root . . . . . . . . . . . . . . . . . ½ pound.
Spikenard Root . . . . . . . . . . . . . . . . . . . ½ pound.
Comfrey Root . . . . . . . . . . . . . . . . . . . . ½ pound.
Mash the roots well, boil in one gallon of water until it is down to a quart, put in a half gallon jug or bottle, add eight ounces of alcohol and a pint and a half of strained honey, or syrup made of sugar. Dose, a teaspoonful every two hours.

## Populus Tremuloides - Poplar

This is a very valuable remedy, and should be used more than it is, and would be if everybody knew of its valuable properties. It is a plant common to this country, and is best gathered in the fall of the year, and is within the reach of everybody.

Medical properties and uses: There are two kinds of barks, white and yellow; one is as good as the other. It is a very valuable remedy in all stomach troubles. It is a fine tonic, and should be used in cases of general debility with feeble digestion. It is good for convalescents when the appetite is deficient. My brother, some few years ago had a severe spell of continued fever. After the fever broke his convalescence was very slow; he had no appetite, and was swarthy, weak, and melancholy; the smell of victuals was that of disgust rather than a pleasure. Our family physician, and a good one, gave him tonics, but without the desired effect. I chanced to be at home at the time, and my mother being alarmed about his condition, asked me if I could recommend anything in our line of practice that would be good for him, give him an appetite and build him up. I recommended equal parts of the inner barks of poplar and dogwood and sarsaparilla root, cut up fine and put in a quart bottle until it was half full, then add whisky till full, and take a large tablespoonful, or a common swallow, before each meal. She did so, he took it, and in four weeks gained fifteen pounds. It immediately increased his appetite, strengthened his nerves, and restored his complexion to its natural color. He now lives twenty miles east of Cincinnati, Clermont county, Ohio.
I will give you an Indian formula still better than the above:
Rattle Root, one part; Prickly Ash Bark, two parts; Poplar Bark, two parts; Sarsaparilla Root, two parts; Dogwood and Wild Cherry, one part.

Fill a quart bottle one-half full of the above finely cut up, and add whisky till full. Dose, from a teaspoonful to a tablespoonful before meals. This will cure rheumatism, give an appetite, strengthen the nerves, and purify your blood.

## Stomach Bitters

### Basic

| | |
|---|---|
| Gentian Root, Ground | ½ ounce. |
| Cinchonia Bark, ground | ½ ounce. |
| Orange Peel, ground | ½ ounce. |
| Cinnamon, ground | 1/4 ounce. |
| Anise Seed, ground | ½ ounce. |
| Coriander Seed, ground | 1/3 ounce. |
| Gum Kino, ground | 1/4 ounce. |
| Alcohol | 1 pint. |
| Water | 4 quarts. |
| Sugar | 1 pound. |

Soak the drugs in the alcohol for one week, pour off the tincture, boil the drugs for a few moments in one quart of water, strain, add the tincture, the rest of the water, and sugar. Then you will have a very pleasant and mild stomach tonic and bitters that will promote digestion and guard your system against malaria or chills. Dose, a common swallow or a wine glass full before each meal and on going to bed.

### Farmer's Bitters

| | |
|---|---|
| Tansy | 1/4 ounce. |
| Crushed Gentian Root | 1 ounce. |
| Pulverized Hydrastis Canadensis | 1 ounce. |
| Anise Seed | ½ ounce. |
| Whisky | 1 quart. |

After standing fourteen days it is ready for use, and will be found to be a fine appetizer and a good stomach tonic, as well as a blood purifier. Dose, a common swallow three or four times a day.

### German Bitters

| | |
|---|---|
| German Chamomile | 2 ounces. |
| Sweet Flag | 2 ounces. |
| Orris Root | 4 ounces. |
| Coriander Seed | 1 ½ ounce. |
| Centaury | 1 ounce. |
| Orange Peel | 3 ounces. |
| Alcohol | 4 pints |
| Water | 4 pints. |
| Sugar | 4 ounces. |

Grind the drugs to a coarse powder, percolate with the alcohol and water, filter, and add the sugar. Dose, a tablespoonful three or four times a day.

### Hop Bitters

| | |
|---|---|
| Hops | 4 ounces. |
| Orange Peel | 2 ounces. |
| Cardamom | 1 drachms. |
| Cloves | ½ drachm. |
| Alcohol | 8 ounces. |
| Sherry Wine | 1 pints. |
| Simple Syrup | 1 pint. |

Grind the drugs, macerate in the alcohol and wine for one week, percolate, add the syrup, and enough water to make one gallon. Dose, a wineglassful three or four times a day.

### Stoughton Bitters

| | |
|---|---|
| Orange Peel, ground | 6 ounces. |
| Gentian Root, ground | 8 ounces. |
| Virginia Snake Root, ground | 1 ½ ounce. |
| American Saffron, ground | ½ ounce. |
| Red Saunders, ground | ½ ounce. |
| Alcohol | 4 pints. |
| Water | 4 pints. |

Mix, macerate fourteen days, filter, and add enough diluted alcohol to make one gallon. Dose, a tablespoonful three times a day before meals.

### Thompson's Eye Water

| | |
|---|---|
| Sulphate of Copper | 10 grains. |
| Sulphate of Zinc | 40 grains. |
| Rose Water | 2 pints. |
| Tincture of Saffron | 4 drachms. |
| Tincture of Camphor | 4 drachms. |

Mix and filter. Drop a few drops in the eyes three or four times a day.

### Cough Syrup

| | |
|---|---|
| Tincture of Squill | 2 ounces. |
| Tincture of Lobelia | 2 ounces. |
| Tincture of Paregoric | 2 ounces. |
| Simple Syrup or Honey | 4 ounces. |

Mix. Dose, from a half to a teaspoonful four or five times a day.

### Boneset, Hops, & Hoarhound Candy

| | |
|---|---|
| Fluid Extract of Boneset | 2 ounces. |
| Tincture of Hops | ½ ounce. |
| Tincture of Blood Root | ½ ounce. |
| Hoarhound Fluid Extract | 1 ounce. |
| White Sugar | 24 ounces. |

Boil the mixture until a drop on a cold plate solidifies or gets hard. Divide while warm into little sticks, and then set it away till cool. This forms a fine candy for colds, coughs, hoarseness, minister's sore throat, and consumption.

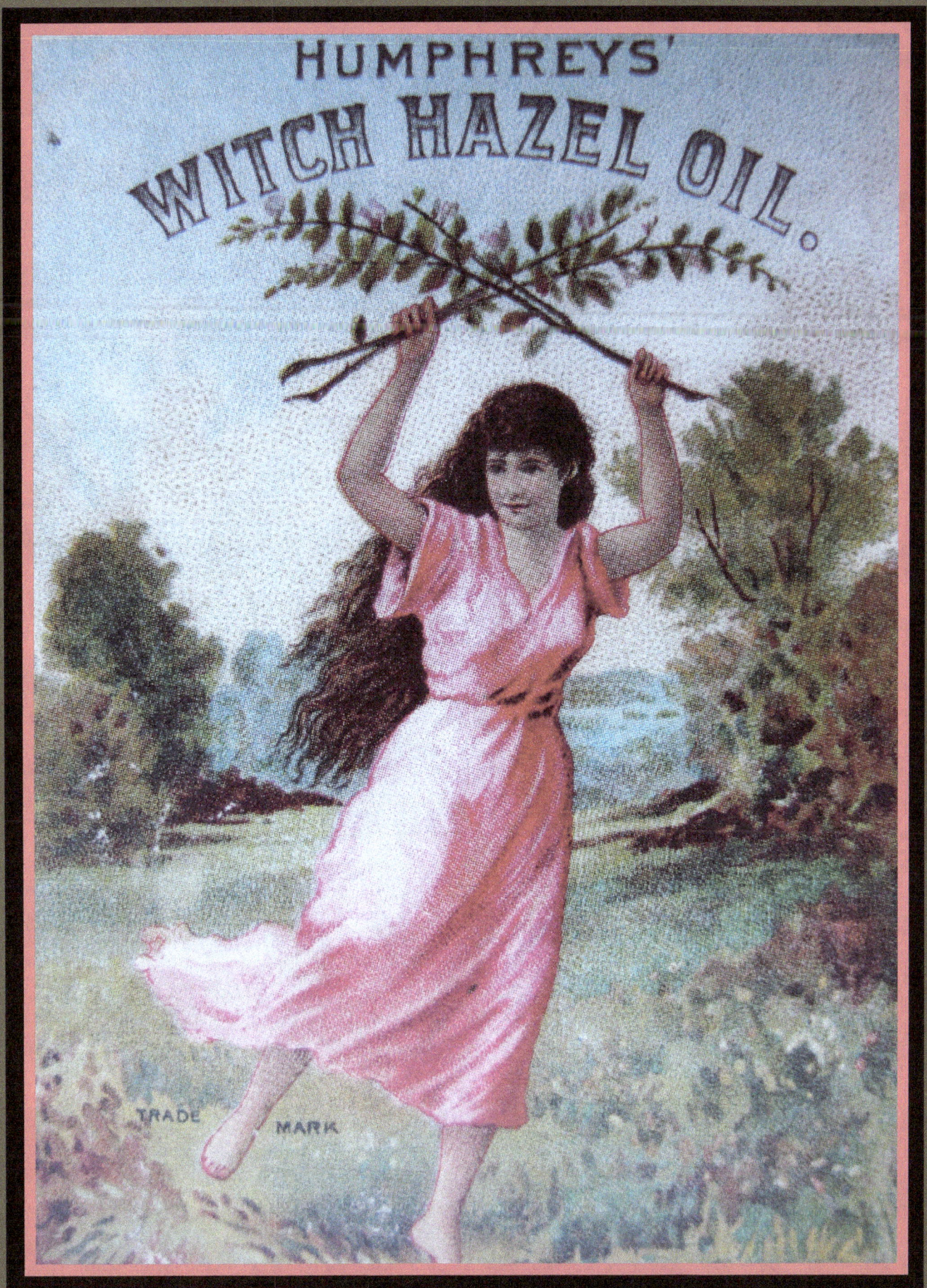

### Act VI

# JOHN HALLECK CENTER
### Folk Herbalist

*John Center was a folk herbalist of the first order, who made his own plant medicines and stood up against the onset of official regulations. He sold his nostrums but treated the poor for free, launching his career with a traveling Medicine Show in 1875, and never quitting until his death at the start of World War II.*

John Halleck Center stood high upon his Medicine Wagon, holding one of his bottles of "botanical wonders" above his head. To the folks gathered to hear his colorful speeches, it may have seemed that this folk herbalist had fashioned his look after the recently deceased gunfighter, Wild Bill Hickok, given his drooping mustache, scarf and wide brimmed "plains" style hat. It was indeed the spirit and lore of the frontier West that inspired him, even though he never in his life ventured far from his Southern Illinois home. He was able to get repeat audiences in the same towns season after season, thanks to the efficacy of some of his nostrums, and the joy of listening to his dramatic histories, exhortations on the amazing flora and fauna of the world, and especially his carefully paced and colorfully delivered rants.

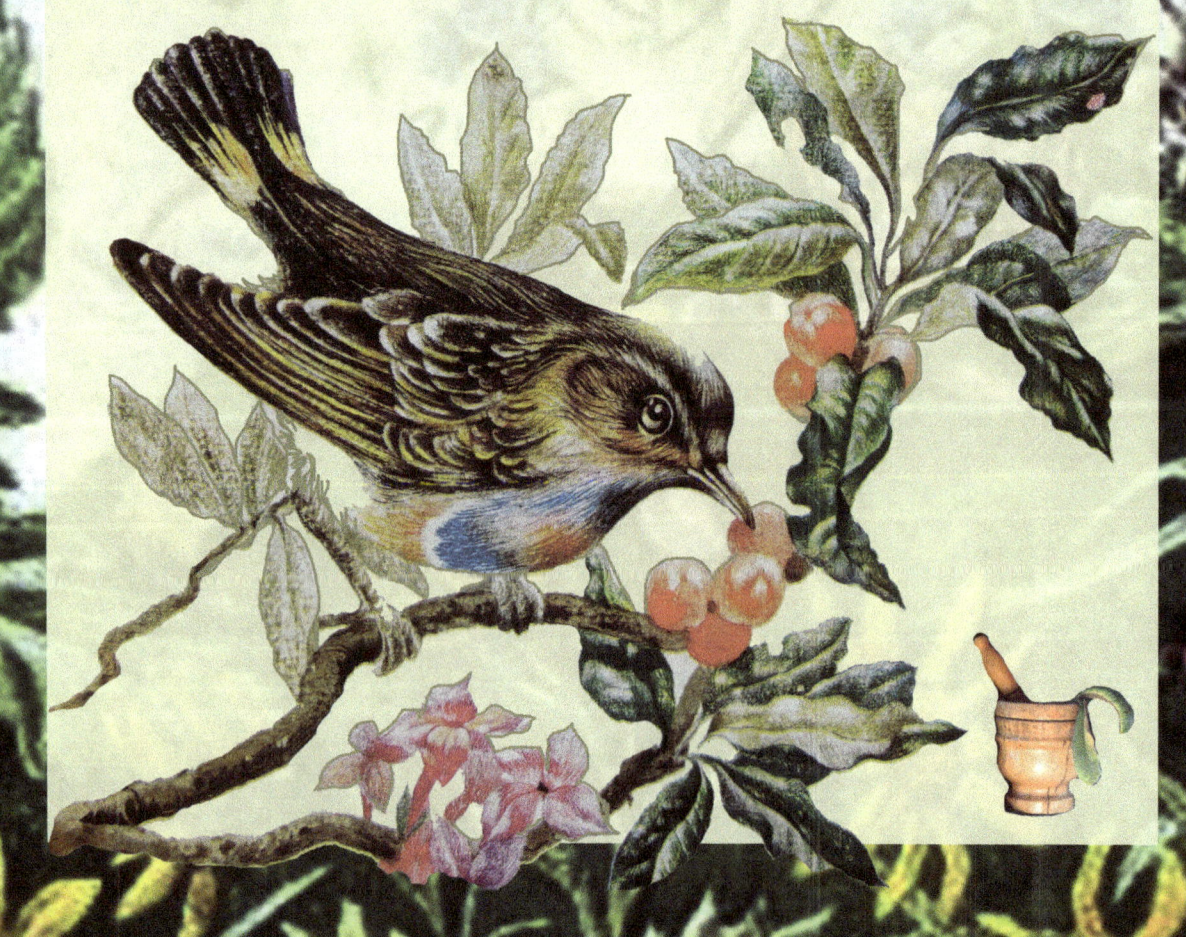

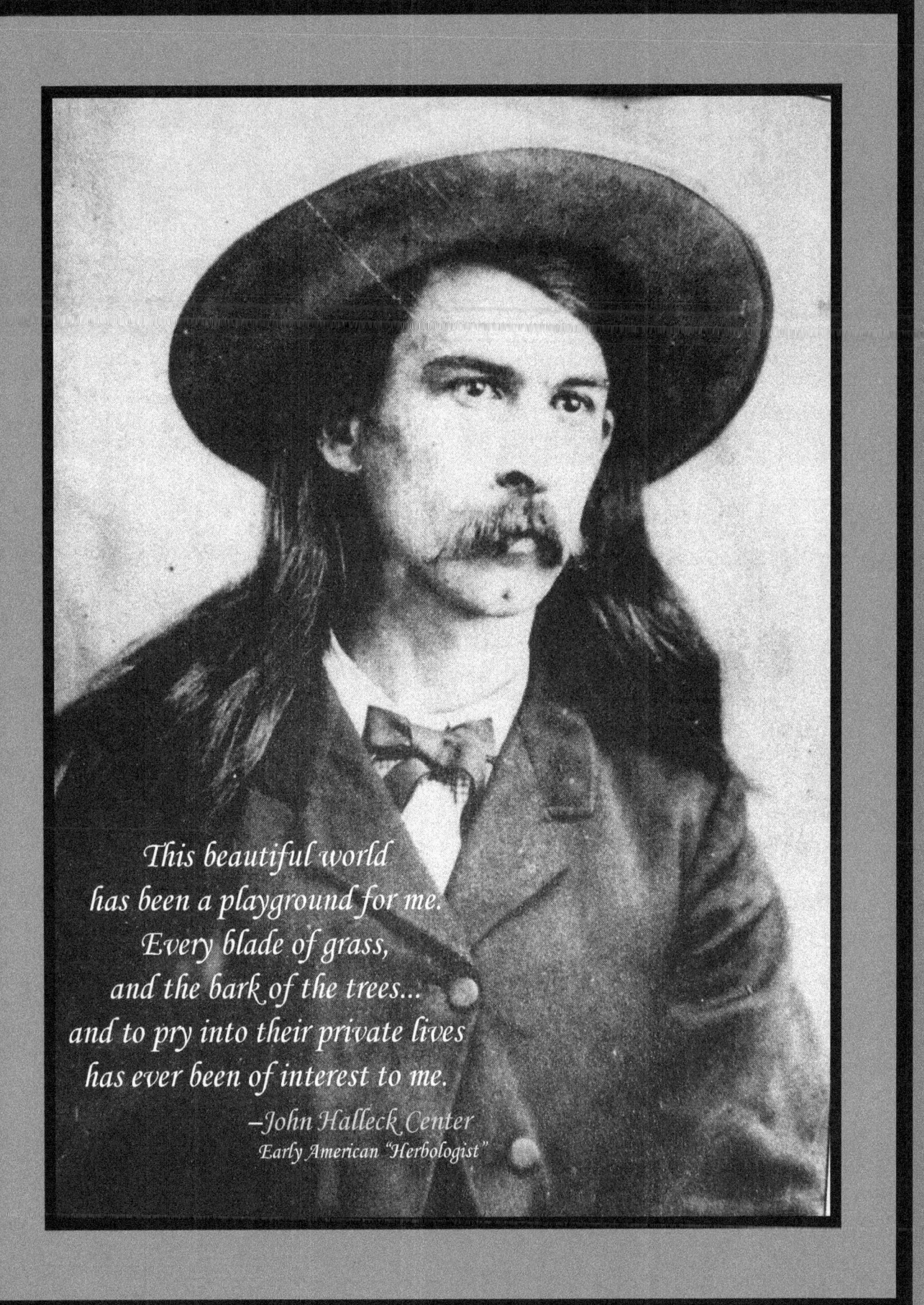

John Halleck preached a brand of earthen mysticism reminiscent of modern strains of Deep Ecology and Animism, touted the benefits of exercise and time spent out in the raw elements and inspiring ferment of nature. His god "would make no hell," he exhorted, as part of a critique of the Old Testament and celebration of the radical ideas of Englishman Charles Darwin. Endangered birds and rare orchids joined medicinal herbs, botany and biology, natural phenomenon and the dangers of government regulation as stimulating topics.

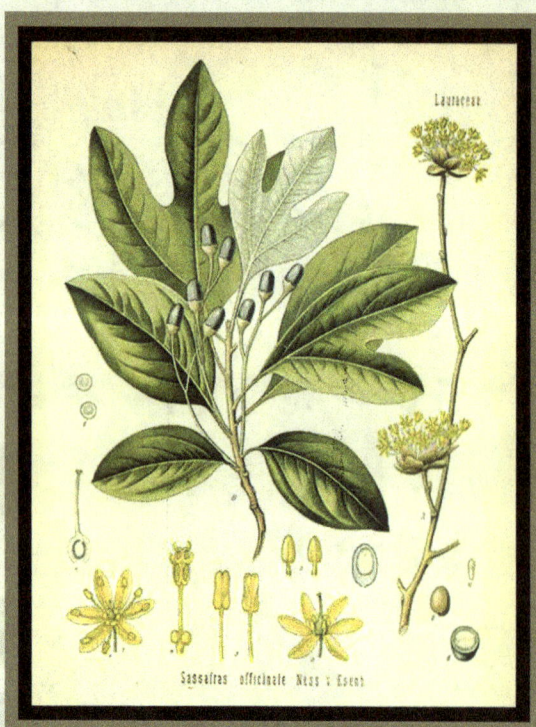

Going against the grain of the times, he railed against the "hypocrisy of the elite," colonialism, the poor treatment of Native Americans by the government, the oppression of women and the plight of underpaid children working in the dangerous underground coal mines that were (and still are) the economic engine of the entire region. And he could, indeed, describe the black dust and drudgery, terror and sweat most intimately, as he had worked what would total more than half a century in those shafts and tunnels himself.

The "grain" that John Halleck went against, was stacked in favor of foreign interventions, male privilege, exploitation of the land as nothing more than lifeless resources, a religiosity of dominion, a loss of self-empowering folk practices, the rising hegemony of so-called "experts" and corporate interests, and what he saw as increasingly less accessible and less affordable health care for the majority of citizens. He always said "and women," anytime he used the word "men," and he insisted on treating Afro-Americans in the face of protests by his white neighbors. Even those who most strongly disagreed with him could regularly be seen assembling for the pleasure of hearing this man speak. It certainly seemed to many that Center cared as much or more about spreading his fiery gospel of natural healing and personal liberation as he did about selling enough medicine to keep himself out of the mines.

Center had grown up with a fascination for all things living, with his childhood room serving as both laboratory and natural history museum, and later his medicine shows garnered extra attention for the collections of animals both preserved and alive, the displays of shells, fossils and carefully pressed and mounted medicinal plants. Apothecary jars filled with enticing flora. A yard-long Mexican iguana with darting tongue. A much discussed diorama of skulls and charts, meant to illustrate and lend evidence to the principles of evolution that he thought it so important to understand. Often joining him were one or more people dressed in traditional Native American garb, usually including his mixed blood wife Josephine billed as the "granddaughter of an Indian medicine woman."

It was from his learned Irish mother Abigail, however, that he got his first herbal education, along with all she knew about taxonomy, astronomy and other fields of wonder. Mrs. Center had augmented her knowledge with the latest medical books, and enlisted young Johnny in the gathering of needed roots and leaves. He would come home from playing with his hair full of various plant parts, and his pockets filled with interesting rocks, bones, and still living creatures. It became a ritual for his mother to stop him at the door, whereupon she would strip him of his cloak of vegetal matter and make him dutifully empty his pockets of any wriggling lizards, rodents or bugs housed therein.

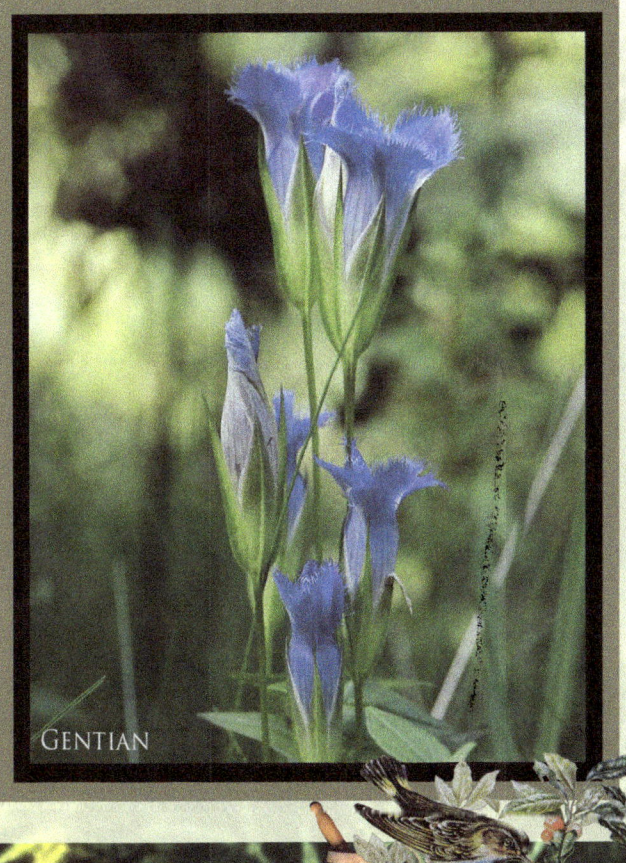
Gentian

The regulation of medicines including homemade herbal preparations begins with the 1906 Food & Drug Act, pushed by the fast growing corporate pharmaceutical industry and passed on a wave of hysteria based on the supposed danger that "patent medicines" posed. John was charged with practicing without a license around this time, convicted on the evidence of his bottle labels with their occasional illegal use of the word "cure," and he had to pay a considerable fine as well as rewrite all his promotional materials.

Due to some medicine sellers falsely promising to cure everything from pimples to cancer with a single decoction, there was some justification for the new rules, but the result has been that honest herbalists from then until now have had to downplay the actual efficacy of the plants we use in order to avoid prosecution. There were relatively few cases of critical harm being done by the bottled remedies being sold, and nothing like the unintended deleterious consequences and long-term side effects of many modern drugs. John Center exemplified the majority of folk herbalists who were committed to offering a safe as well as effective natural remedies. He avoided using alcohol in his preparations whenever possible. And while addictive cocaine and opium were some of the most common ingredients in commercial preparations from the major pharmaceutical companies up until 1914, Center rejected incorporating them into any of his recipes, actively campaigning against their use.

What his medicines did contain included herbs currently accepted as having credible medicinal use, such as Sassafras, Gentian, Fennel, Ginger, Blue Flag, and Queen of The Meadow. He sold untold capsules of Buchu that many consider to be helpful in cases of urinary tract issues. For Bronchitis, he recommended herbs like Aloe and Black Cherry bark, along with virus inhibiting Licorice. A skin balm of Acacia and zinc sulphate. Kamala to rid the system of tapeworms. His most famous product, "Liveon," contained an extract of rhubarb still considered to be a digestive and liver stimulant as well as a strong laxative.

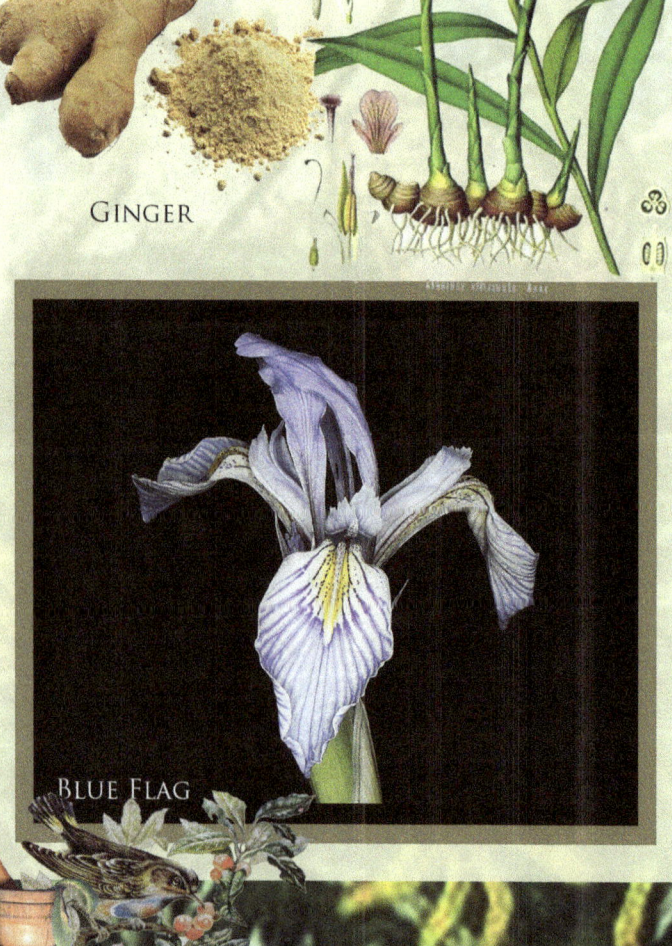

GINGER

BLUE FLAG

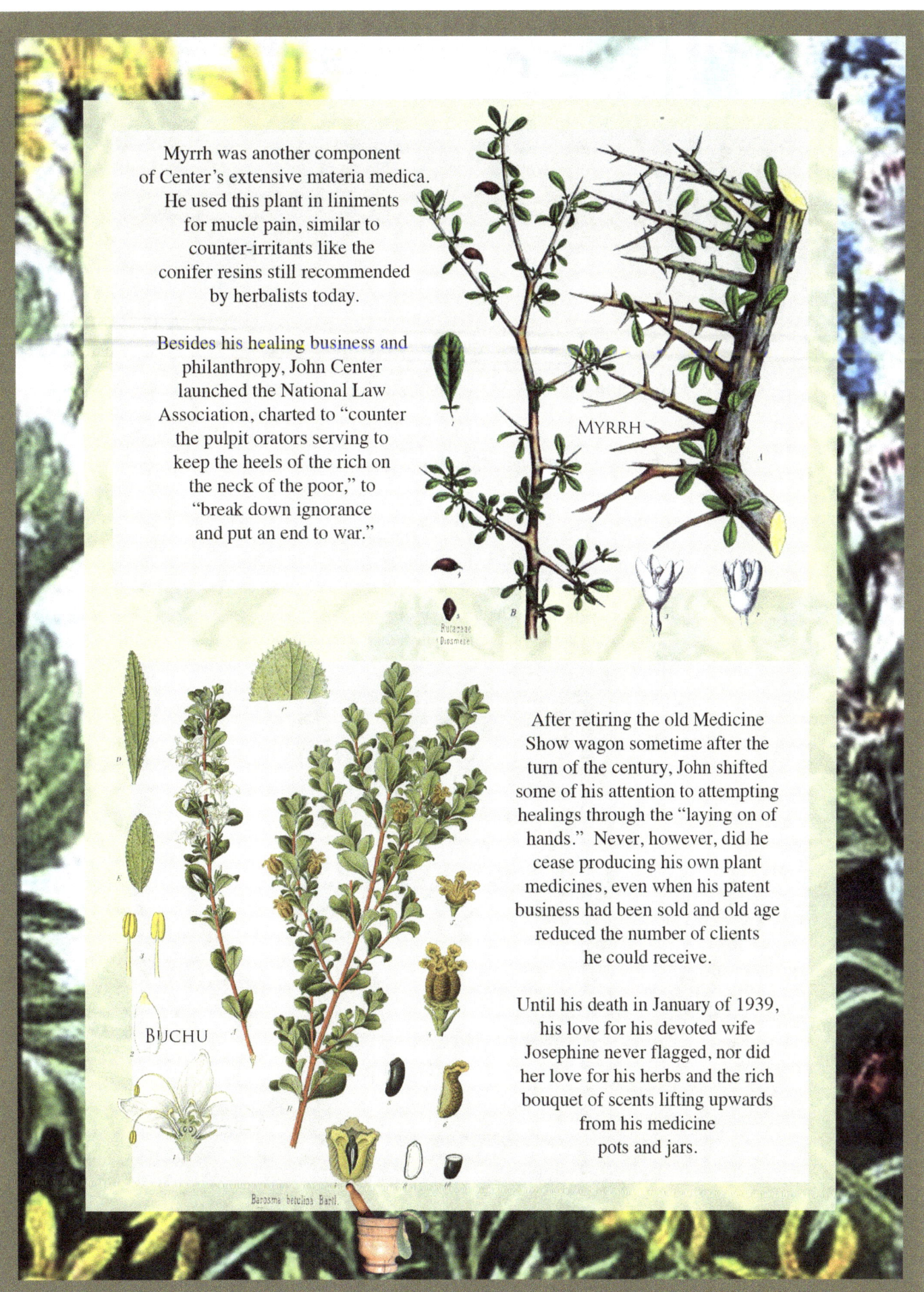

Myrrh was another component of Center's extensive materia medica. He used this plant in liniments for mucle pain, similar to counter-irritants like the conifer resins still recommended by herbalists today.

Besides his healing business and philanthropy, John Center launched the National Law Association, charted to "counter the pulpit orators serving to keep the heels of the rich on the neck of the poor," to "break down ignorance and put an end to war."

After retiring the old Medicine Show wagon sometime after the turn of the century, John shifted some of his attention to attempting healings through the "laying on of hands." Never, however, did he cease producing his own plant medicines, even when his patent business had been sold and old age reduced the number of clients he could receive.

Until his death in January of 1939, his love for his devoted wife Josephine never flagged, nor did her love for his herbs and the rich bouquet of scents lifting upwards from his medicine pots and jars.

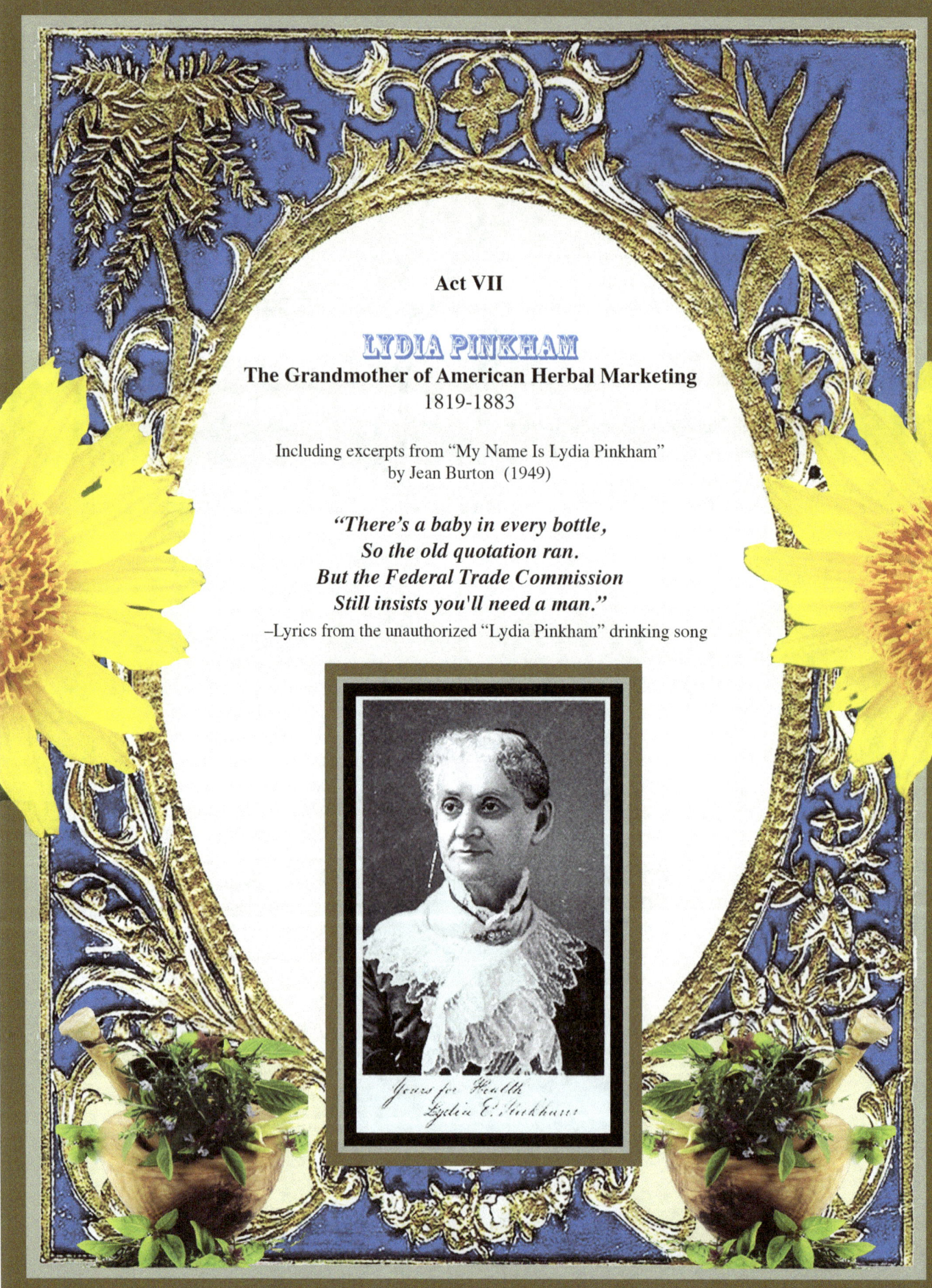

### Act VII

## LYDIA PINKHAM
**The Grandmother of American Herbal Marketing**
1819-1883

Including excerpts from "My Name Is Lydia Pinkham"
by Jean Burton (1949)

*"There's a baby in every bottle,
So the old quotation ran.
But the Federal Trade Commission
Still insists you'll need a man."*
–Lyrics from the unauthorized "Lydia Pinkham" drinking song

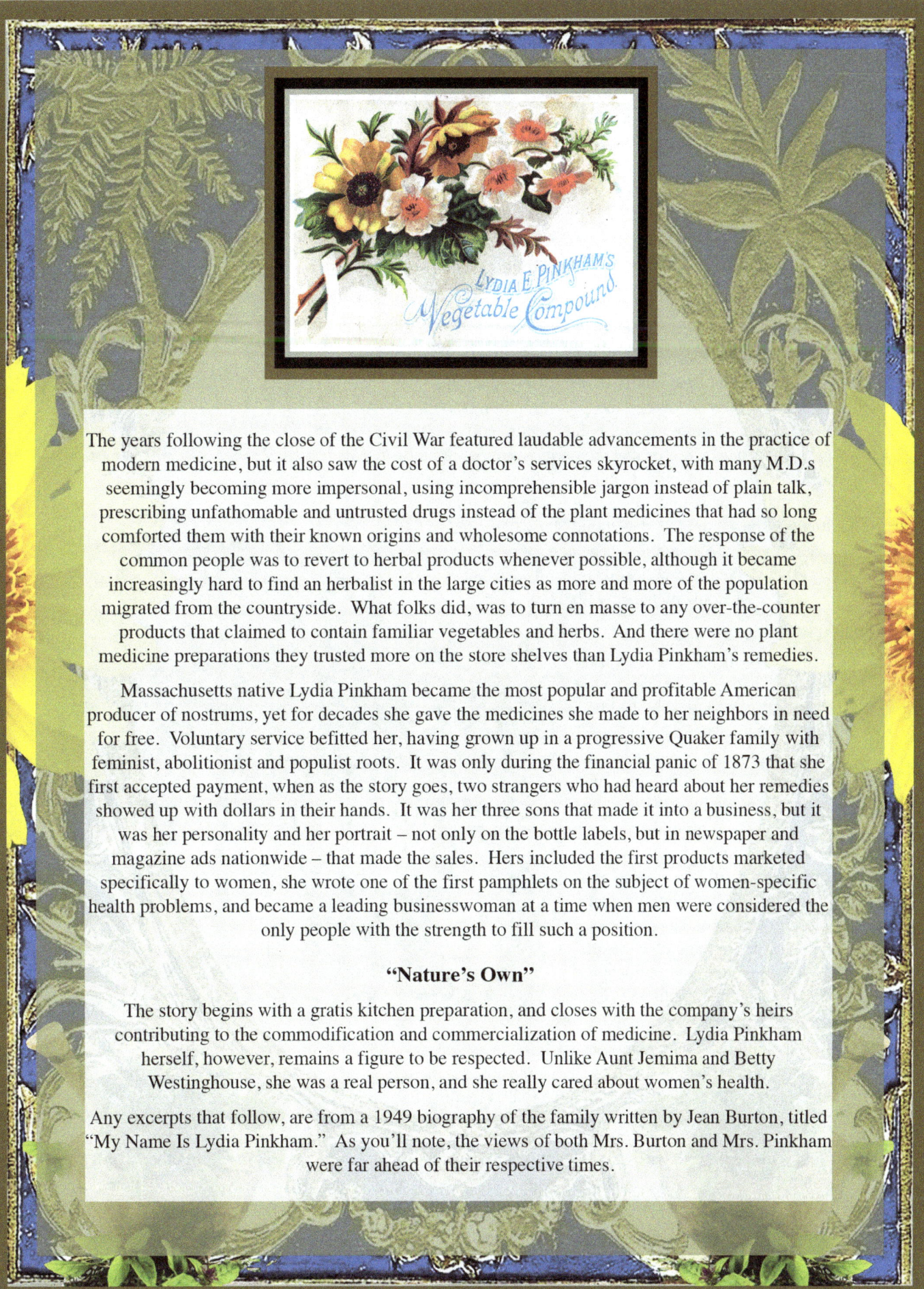

The years following the close of the Civil War featured laudable advancements in the practice of modern medicine, but it also saw the cost of a doctor's services skyrocket, with many M.D.s seemingly becoming more impersonal, using incomprehensible jargon instead of plain talk, prescribing unfathomable and untrusted drugs instead of the plant medicines that had so long comforted them with their known origins and wholesome connotations. The response of the common people was to revert to herbal products whenever possible, although it became increasingly hard to find an herbalist in the large cities as more and more of the population migrated from the countryside. What folks did, was to turn en masse to any over-the-counter products that claimed to contain familiar vegetables and herbs. And there were no plant medicine preparations they trusted more on the store shelves than Lydia Pinkham's remedies.

Massachusetts native Lydia Pinkham became the most popular and profitable American producer of nostrums, yet for decades she gave the medicines she made to her neighbors in need for free. Voluntary service befitted her, having grown up in a progressive Quaker family with feminist, abolitionist and populist roots. It was only during the financial panic of 1873 that she first accepted payment, when as the story goes, two strangers who had heard about her remedies showed up with dollars in their hands. It was her three sons that made it into a business, but it was her personality and her portrait – not only on the bottle labels, but in newspaper and magazine ads nationwide – that made the sales. Hers included the first products marketed specifically to women, she wrote one of the first pamphlets on the subject of women-specific health problems, and became a leading businesswoman at a time when men were considered the only people with the strength to fill such a position.

### "Nature's Own"

The story begins with a gratis kitchen preparation, and closes with the company's heirs contributing to the commodification and commercialization of medicine. Lydia Pinkham herself, however, remains a figure to be respected. Unlike Aunt Jemima and Betty Westinghouse, she was a real person, and she really cared about women's health.

Any excerpts that follow, are from a 1949 biography of the family written by Jean Burton, titled "My Name Is Lydia Pinkham." As you'll note, the views of both Mrs. Burton and Mrs. Pinkham were far ahead of their respective times.

*From the book:*

"Doctors in the 1850s and 60s relied chiefly on bleeding, blistering, cupping and leeching. For internal medicine they leaned heaviest on vermifuges, nux vomica (strychnine), opium, quinine, antimony and calomel. Calomel in particular – a mixture of metallic mercury and corrosive sublimate – was the favored cure-all, routinely pre-scribed for nearly every complaint and in alarming quantities. If a patient did not feel better after an ounce of calomel had passed through his system, he was urged to try another ounce without delay. As one result, there were people in every community who had developed the unpleasant symptoms of mercury poisoning in the course of treatment. As another result, public sentiment became aggrieved to such a degree that the daily press, beginning with more or less restrained allusions to quacks, robbers and humbugs, worked up to a point where doctors were habitually referred to almost as though they belonged in the category of public enemies. The newspapers prided themselves on outspokenness, and were not inconvenienced by libel laws.

In the 1850s and 60s, when various schools of medical reformers began to be heard from, they launched their concerted attack on the old materia medica with all the fanfare of a new political movement, complete with national conventions, lecture tours, open debates and official propaganda organs. The public, on its part, took sides vehemently; in a democratic society it was felt that one man's opinion was as good as another's, in medicine or anything else. Besides, these movements had philosophic, sociological and nationalistic overtones.

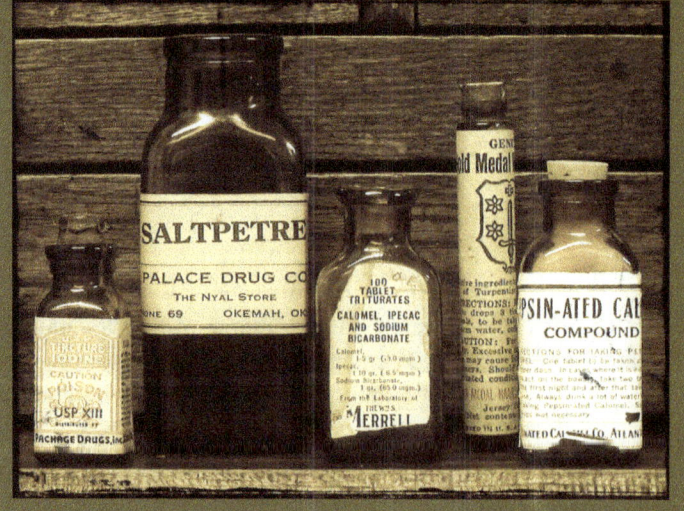

Hitherto there had not been much original research to which Americans could point with pride, and they found it intolerable that medicine should remain in a humble state of colonial dependence. Dr. Holmes himself was not immune to this feeling; he complained that medical writers in the United States were simply 'putting British portraits of disease in American frames'.

What Lydia believed, was that: 'The most judicious help of all was Nature's own', in other words, botanic remedies. As Mrs. Pinkham came to say of her Compound, "It will at all times and under all circumstances act in harmony with the laws that govern the female system.'

The greatest contribution of the Eclectics was their investigation of the therapeutic value of native plants. The fact that they were native plants was a good deal stressed; their vegetable and herb drugs were recommended as being not only efficacious, but as possessing the further virtue of being 100% American.

This fell agreeably on the public ear; it was something most people were familiar with. Lynn, a fairly representative community in this respect, could still remember the self-sufficient era when families not only made their own clothes, carpets, quilts, furniture, candles and soap, but also attended to their own first-aid and doctoring. A physician was not called in till all other means had failed. Every good housewife kept on hand a store of 'simples' (for external application) and 'medicinals' prepared from roots, leaves and herbs. The recipes for some of these had been brought from England by the first Puritans, and dated back heaven knows how far. As time went on the settlers learned the uses of various local vegetable drugs from the Indians.

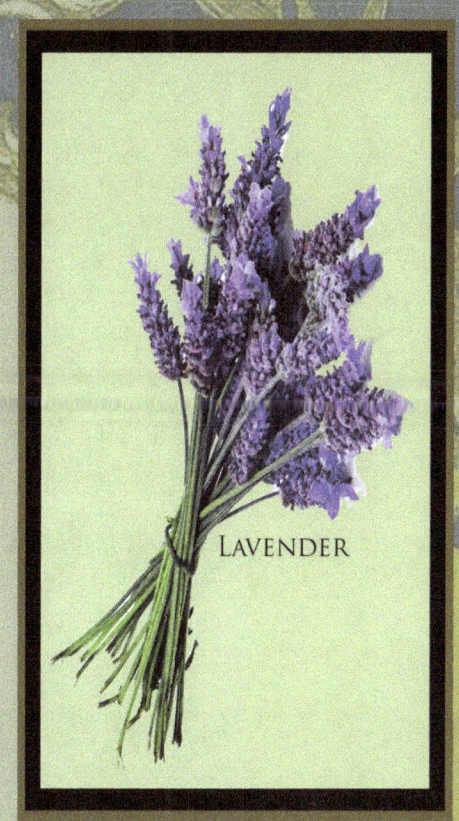

LAVENDER

Mrs. Pinkham herself had grown up in a farmhouse where the attic was always pungent with dried thyme, mint, lavender and mandrake, gathered in spring and fall. Everyone knew that colds were best treated with boneset tea, mullein, tansy or bugleweed. Fevers called for vervain and monkshood. For aches and pains, witch-hazel, arnica or garget-berry were indicated; for indigestion, wintergreen or spearmint. Wild indigo relieved sore eyes. Infusion of foxglove was used for heart trouble centuries before the discovery that it contained digitalis.

Of the many volumes written by leaders of the Eclectic School, the one that struck Mrs. Pinkham as most eminently sensible was The American Dispensatory, by Dr. John King of Cincinnati. King is remembered today chiefly as a pioneer pharmacologist, the first to isolate the active principles of numerous plants and introduce them into medical practice. The apparatus he evolved for this purpose, primitive but ingenious, may be seen in the Smithsonian Institution at Washington.

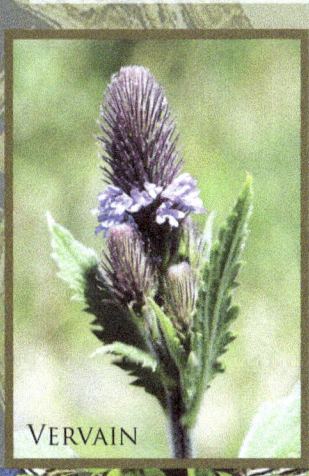

VERVAIN

The American Dispensatory, a massive compendium of botanic lore, went through eighteen editions in his lifetime. Its preamble stated a point of view that Lydia found strongly sympathetic. 'A large class of physicians in America,' asserted Dr. King, 'believe that the profession has been too much trammeled by the influence of Authority...
The assumption of infallibility in the existing and prevalent system of Therapeutics is too extravagant to bear the test of serious examination. No one point is more universally denied by the American people than the exclusive right of one set of men to judge and have sole control in any thing. Persecution or proscription for opinion's sake is not tolerated in political or religious matters; and certainly should not be in those pertaining to medicine.'

## Pinkham's Famous Vegetable Compound

The section of the Dispensatory that caught Mrs. Pinkham's eye dealt with Aletris farinosa or, as it was popularly and more colorfully known, True Unicorn, a bitter-rooted herb which in the long history of vegetable drugs had been somewhat puzzlingly described as both a uterine tonic and a uterine sedative. It had been used since the earliest recorded days of Indian medicine, which gave rise later to a widespread belief that the Vegetable Compound was based on 'an old squaw remedy' Perhaps indirectly it was, for Dr. King spent considerable time enthusiastically tracking down rumors of authentic Indian cures. At any rate he thought highly of Aletris, whether administered alone or in combination with extract of Asclepias (Pleurisy Root). The effects of this latter were so pronounced that Dr. King did not care to commit himself as to just how important a discovery he might have happened upon. 'In uterine difficulties,' he stated cautiously, 'this plant deserves further investigation. It is, undoubtedly, one of our most useful agents.'

The original formula, if anyone had cared to go out in the dark of the moon and gather his own supply of the needful herbs, called for:
8 oz. True Unicorn Root
8 oz. False Unicorn Root
6 oz. Life Root
6 oz. Black Cohosh
6 oz. Pleurisy Root
12 oz. Fenugreek Seed

There was never any secrecy about the ingredients, nor yet about the way they were prepared. In the early days the company went to considerable expense to describe each step in some detail, which was also a revolutionary departure. They simply thought that people would be interested, and they were right. Mrs. Pinkham bought her roots and herbs already dried and ground, so they could be weighed on kitchen balances or measured in a cup. Some were steeped, some soaked in cold water, some macerated in dilute alcohol Then they were mixed all together and percolated through cloth.

Mrs. Pinkham embarked on this business innocent of the very slightest knowledge of pharmacy or laboratory methods. The first operations, in consequence, were a good deal more like cooking than chemistry. A cellar kitchen, immaculately scrubbed out and set in readiness, was reserved for this purpose. Penetrating aromatic scents floated up daily to the family kitchen and living rooms on the floor above. In the evenings the assembled family would bottle the day's supply. The bottles were then packed for shipment in second-hand boxes procured from a nearby grocer.

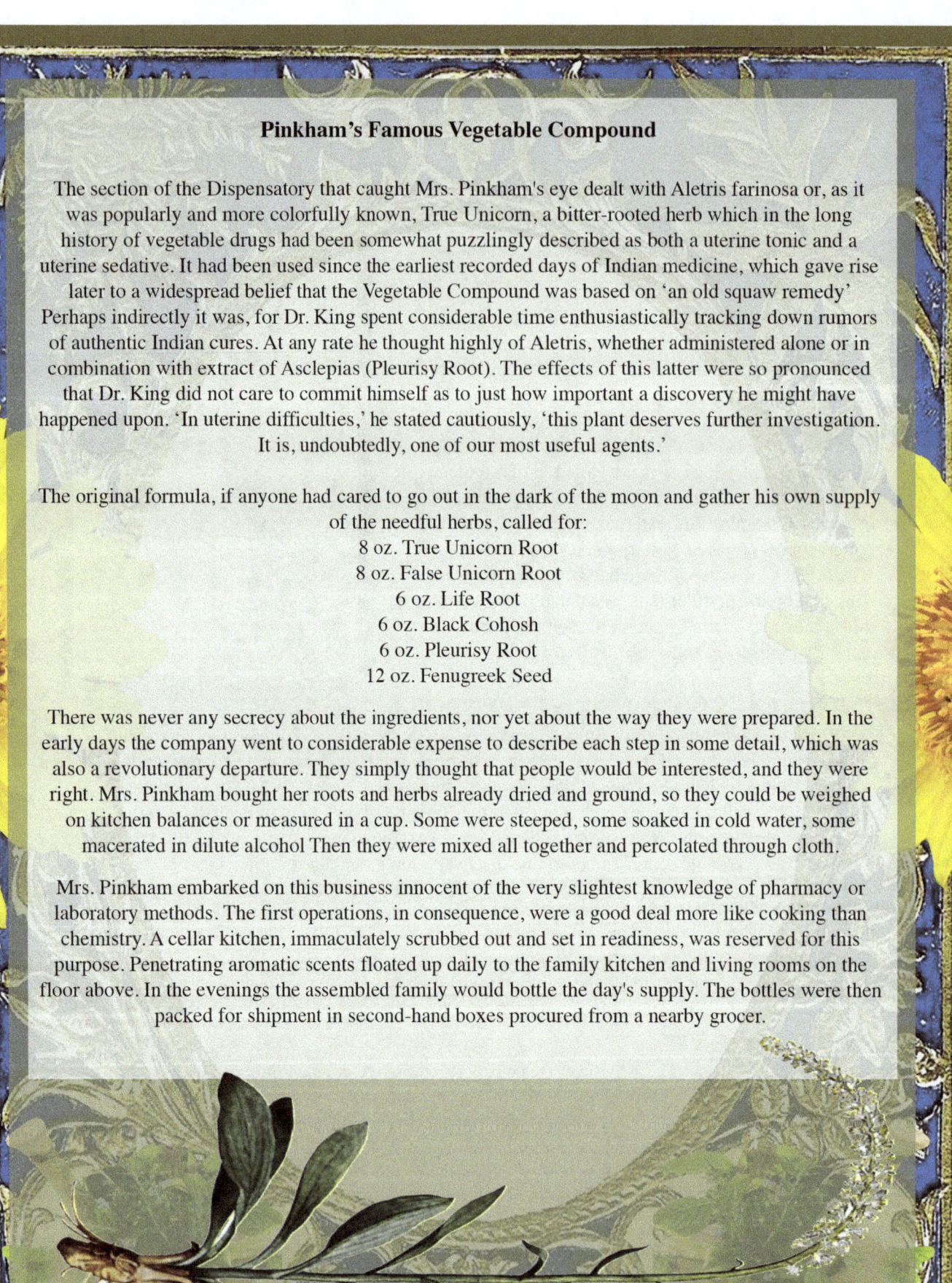

Unicorn Root

## Herbal Marketing

Whatever the efficacy of Pinkham's compounds, the reasons they became the leading proprietary (so called "patent") medicines of the day had mostly to do with her persona, and the ways she constantly and personally reached out to her mostly female customers.

"Mrs. Pinkham wrote copy for the handbills herself, plus for the labels and their first four-page pamphlet entitled Guide for Women. She had to improvise as she went along, but from the first her tone was assured; she knew just how to catch and hold a woman's interest. And this was a matter to which advertisers hitherto had given scant thought, no doubt feeling that the purchasing power represented by butter-and-egg money was not enough to inspire any great effort.

Confidence in this line came naturally to Mrs. Pinkham who, though she might speak deprecatingly of herself as 'an untitled woman who has no higher ambition than to do good for others', had for years possessed a unique formula, a complete medical theory to explain it, and an articulately grateful local following.

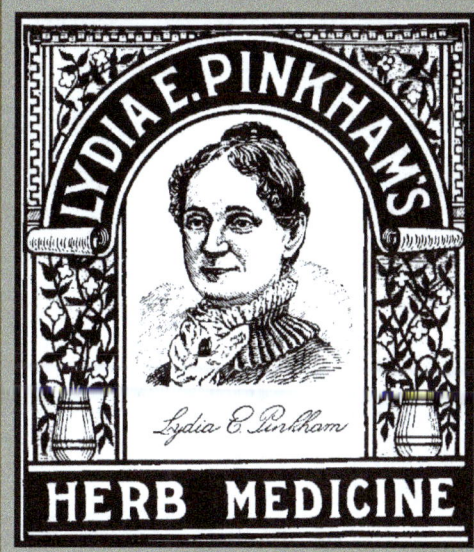

"Mrs. Pinkham naturally found it pleasurable to see the sales curve rise, this being impersonal. But to the end of her days she never got over feeling a distinct awkwardness about taking money from people she knew; and many people insisted on making the trip to Lynn to consult her in person. The next step might have been foreseen in the nature of things, 'Write to Mrs. Pinkham at Lynn, Mass., and she will advise you,' every advertisement cordially urged. From the time of Lydia's death in 1883 until they were finally exposed some 20 years later, the company run by her disingenuous offspring continued to send out individualized replies to the many anxious women, each purporting to be signed by Mrs. Pinkham herself, and with every reply including a recommendation that they try using certain of their products. Yet for as long as she lived, Lydia insisted on personally answering all of the letters that came in, albeit with the help of her "lady" stenographers.

### LYDIA E. PINKHAM'S HERB MEDICINE

Lydia E. Pinkham's Herb Medicine is a reliable general tonic, equally good for men and women. It takes the place of Grandma's sulphur and molasses in the Spring and is much more pleasant to the taste. Keep it in the medicine chest and give it to the whole family—parents and children—at any time through the year when they need such a medicine.

A new photograph was the next thing indicated. The result was absolutely inspired to the last detail, the neat black silk dress, the tortoise-shell comb, the white face fichu fastened with a cameo brooch. It was worth every penny of the 40 million dollars subsequently spent on keeping her image before the public eye. Mrs. Pinkham's elderly features, handsome, sagacious and composed, were those of everybody's dream grandmother."

# LYDIA E. PINKHAM'S
## PRIVATE TEXT-BOOK

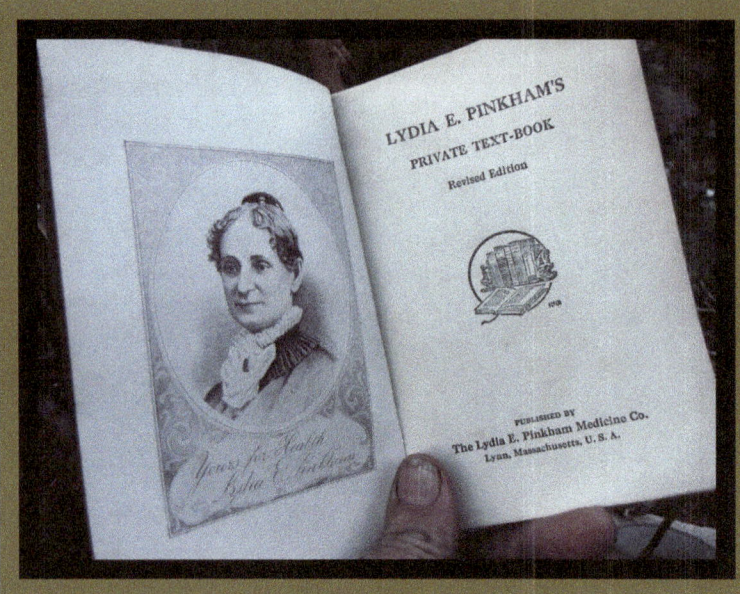

PUBLISHED BY
### The Lydia E. Pinkham Medicine Co.
Lynn, Massachusetts, U. S. A.

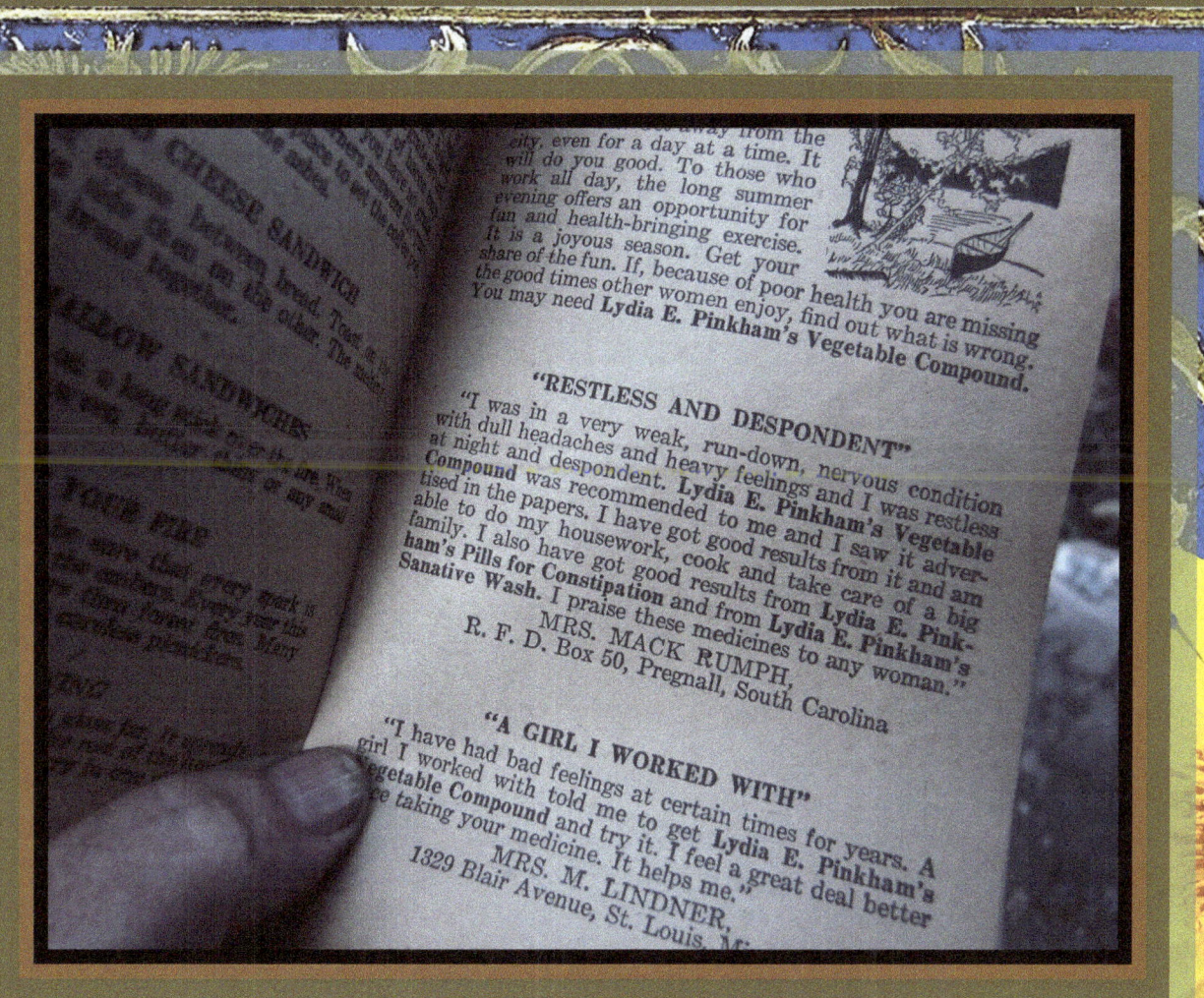

## Advice From Lydia

"Mrs. Pinkham's basic rules for health represented for whole sections of the public positively their first introduction to the principles of hygiene. Above all she campaigned for elementary cleanliness 'Keep clean inside and out!' and attacked the widespread prejudice against fresh air, particularly night air: 'Ventilate! Ventilate! Ventilate! Sleep with open windows!' (She did not go so far as to recommend a room of one's own, but she did say that it would add years to most women's lives if they could get away from their families just for one blessed hour of privacy out of the twenty-four.)

Diet reform was another of her concerns. In view of the kind and quantity of food generally consumed, it was small wonder that anti-bilious pills were in dire demand. Entire communities were accustomed to subsist through the winter months on a diet of beans, salt pork and doughnuts. The Grahamites declared grimly that vast numbers of their fellow-Americans were in a chronically toxic condition as the result of sheer gluttony, recording their further conviction that a hundred thousand fatalities each year might be attributed to this cause alone. Mrs. Pinkham could not see quite eye to eye with them in their vegetarian crusade, but she joined them in urging the use of whole grain cereals, bran and plenty of fresh fruits and vegetables. A typical letter included the injunction: 'Eat no pastry nor fine Flour, but Graliain bread, the various mushes and fruit. Ride out, walk out, dig, use the trowel Study the hygienic laws that your own nature requires'.

As both sexes suffered lamentably from dyspepsia 'the symptoms,' mused Mrs. Pinkham 'include great distress at pit of stomach, heaviness or burning sensation, causing the patient to feel melancholy and at times morose. A general sense of discomfort seems to pervade the entire system. For relief, try':

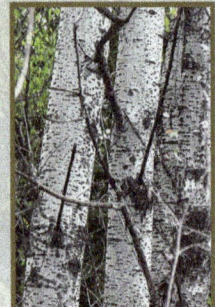
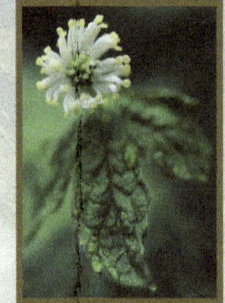

1 Ib Wild Poplar Bark
4 oz. Golden Seal
4 oz. Gentian Root
3 oz. Cinchona (Peruvian Bark)
2 oz. Cardamon Seeds (a stomachic)
4 oz. Camomile Flowers
Refined Cayenne Pepper

The whole percolated in 1 gal. of best spirits with water and sugar added.

'The above if persisted in will perform a cure in the most obstinate cases if taken in proper doses and pork of all kinds and salt fish avoided, also any food that tends to create wind.'

Note that she freely shared her medicine recipes, rather than just pushing for product sales. For example, advice in her letters to sufferers included, to one: "White pine hark is good for sluggish kidneys." And to a woman with an aching back she suggested simply that "If taken with great distress in the back, apply a bag of salt heated hot'. Nor were her suggestions always the most credible, since like many in the alternative medicine field, her hopefulness and enthusiasm had her also buying into less helpful superstitions ('For a sure cure for hiccoughs, place a bag of hops upon the pit of the stomach') as well as the latest if health fads from magnetic belts to electric therapy. Impressively, the recognized the impact of the psyche and attitude or preconception on symptoms and suffering, telling one correspondent that her 'symptoms supposed to be indications of malarial trouble are probably the result of nervous prostration' instead.

Lydia's political sense of the empowered woman was in synch with her views on the female constitution. As Jean Burton points out:

"Pinkham had not the slightest use for the cult of fragility – which in any case, as she was in a position to know, had far fewer adherents than he might have supposed from contemplation of the wasp-waisted belles in Godey's Magazine. A fashionable clergyman might, as in the widely quoted funeral sermon for one Susanna Pierce, list among the winsome attributes of the deceased a 'constitutional delicacy of organization' which had imparted to her features 'that peculiar charm which no healthful comeliness can ever confer,' but Mrs. Pinkham was well aware that to the great mass of ordinary women with families to feed and floors to scrub, not to mention underpaid factory girls and hard-driven farm wives, such charm appeared peculiar indeed. As for the theory that feminine appeal was synonymous with helplessness, Mrs, Pinkham contented herself with observing briefly: *'Weakness Is Never the Source of Power'*.

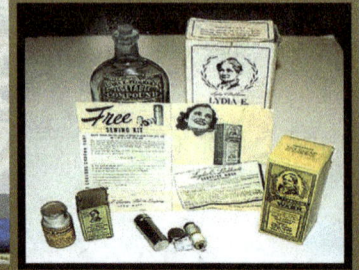

# Relations With the Medical Establishment

"At this period the relations between the Compound's discoverer and the medical establishment might be described as wary, but not always or openly antagonistic. Mrs. Pinkham often stressed that 'Physicians Use It and Prescribe It Freely', evidently intending this to be construed in its favor. And it was a fact, particularly in the case of older doctors who had been using botanicals all their professional lives. Druggists till around the turn of the century often ordered a supply of the Compound in gallon lots, so that it could be dispensed on prescription, an indication that this was fairly routine procedure.

Yet the element of rivalry was always implicit. Mrs. Pinkham looked tolerantly upon doctors when they were prescribing her Compound but not, on the whole, otherwise. They were credited with good intentions, and that was about all.

On general principles, she felt similarly skeptical regarding medical diagnosis; particularly in the field of gynecology, which admittedly, in her day, could hardly be called a dependable science. 'In certain diseases' she allowed, 'the scientific physician, with the aid of the microscope, etc., may be enabled to give an accurate diagnosis; but with the patient:, the remedy is the thing.'

Pinkham kept a voluminous casebook, dated 1878 on the flyleaf, to record her own diagnoses and recommendations, and often were at variance with those of orthodox practitioners, such as when she wrote that people had for too long 'taken virulent poisons in the form of medicine.'

For several years after the Compound first came on the market, Pinkham's sons promoted it for virtually every known disability, up to and including a prolapsed uterus. Her ingenious theory was that it so strengthened and toned the ligaments supporting this organ that it would gradually resume its normal position. Inexplicably, customers often assured her that it had performed this feat, thereby confirming her faith in its magic over-all potency. In point of fact, there were only two conditions in which it was useful for menstrual difficulties and it was 50 years after her death before anyone knew how or why.

# Legal Challenges

As far back as 1892, the editor of the Ladies' Home Journal had refused to accept further patent medicine advertisements, and had gone on to indict a long list of products, freely purchasable in any state, as doped or otherwise dangerous. Samuel Hopkins Adams had followed with the sensational revelations of The Great American Fraud. In 1913, partly as a result of these campaigns, broad powers over labeling were given to the Federal Food and Drug Administration; and in 1914 the Federal Trade Commission was empowered to deal with unfair trade practices, including fraudulent claims in advertising.

So far the Compound had been little affected. In 1914 the formula was somewhat changed; dandelion and yellow gentian, the base of the bitter Swiss cordial, were added, but the main ingredients remained the same. About a year later the alcohol content was reduced to 15 per cent. The only result the company noticed was that sales soared as never before. They were also fortunate in that the new regulations had not forced them to discard one of their greatest assets, the time-honored name of their principal product. A Vegetable Compound was what the label said, and a Vegetable Compound it indubitably was. Finally, even when the nationwide campaign against the "Poison Trust" had been at its height, the harshest critics of the Compound had never claimed that it did its users any actual harm. What they did assert was that it did no one any particular good, either; and that misguided women who depended on it might put off medical treatment till too late. In 1921 the American Medical Association in its historic Nostrums and Quackery disposed of the Compound by citing an earlier analysis by volume made by chemists of the British Medical Association, showing it to contain so much alcohol, so much ash, solid matter, and vegetable extractive matter. But they had not tested the latter for any possible efficacy, stating that it 'possessed no distinctive characteristics.'

Near the end of 1925 the company encountered its first serious trouble with the authorities. The Food and Drug Administration formally objected to the wording on the Compound package. Though much less comprehensive in its claims than it had once been, it still covered a good deal of territory. At the factory all operations were suspended till new packages could be obtained, and employees worked straight through Christmas Day rewrapping bottles. Under the new dispensation the Compound was 'Recommended as a vegetable tonic in conditions for which this preparation is adapted,' whatever those might be.

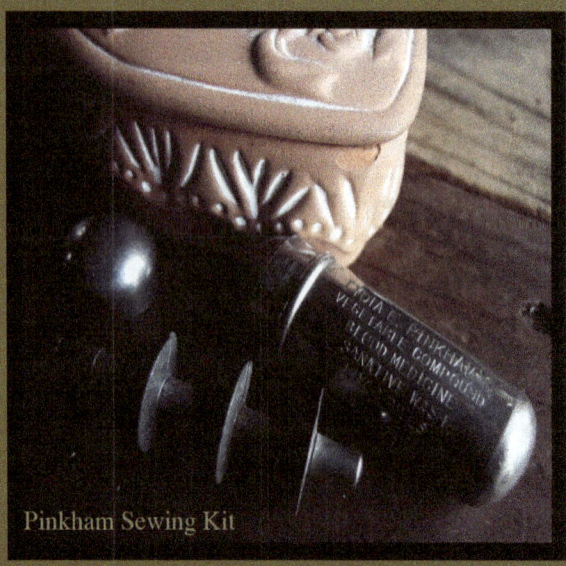

Pinkham Sewing Kit

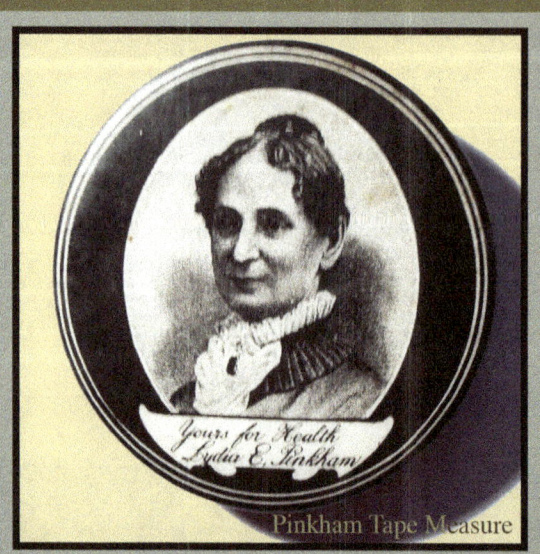

Pinkham Tape Measure

Matters rested here for some ten years, till in 1938 they faced imminent catastrophe. The Food and Drug Administration sent to the Federal Trade Commission its 'Scientific Opinion' that the Compound was at best a mild stomachic tonic, and as such of no more benefit to women than to men. Two years earlier this pronouncement might have been fatal; but on the strength of new research undertaken, the company was in a much stronger position. The Federal Trade Commission sent a copy of this 'opinion' to the company, and negotiations were begun.

After more than two years, with protracted hearings in Washington, the Federal Trade Commission and the company signed a stipulation, as a result of which the company was free to continue and to press its advertising claim that the Compound was indeed a uterine sedative.

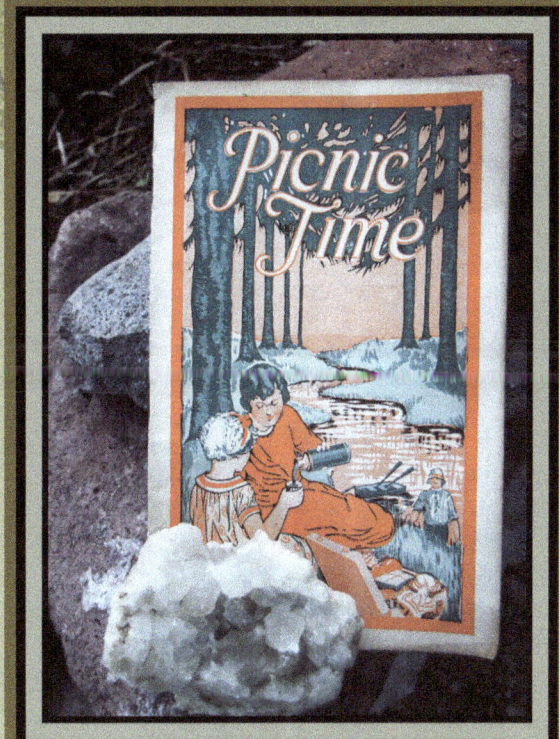

One curious disclosure was that there appear to be cycles of fashion even in drugs. Two of the drugs on which the Compound mainly depended, Aletris (True Unicorn) and Asclepias (Pleurisy Root) had not only passed completely out of fashion but were almost forgotten, having been dropped from the United States Pharmacopoeia for over forty years. As for the Compound as a whole, the findings were that when administered in the treatment of patients during the climacteric syndrome, it markedly decreased the number of vasomotor disturbances experienced each day (or as Mrs. Pinkham would have put it, women had fewer hot flushes when going through the Change); and that with patients who experienced menstrual pain severe enough to send them to clinics for relief, it appeared to 'establish a normal rhythm in a previously arhythmic contractile pattern, and to eliminate superimposed contractions on the normal contractile phase.'

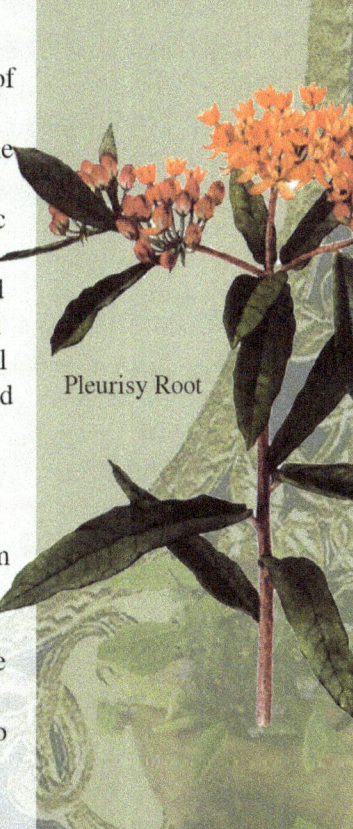

Pleurisy Root

The general reaction to this was intense surprise. Mrs. Pinkham would have experienced no such emotion, though she might have felt serenely gratified to learn that science had at length caught up with her. After all, she had thought highly of science at a time when the neighbors did not. Her Compound could hardly do all that she had believed it capable of, but it could do one or two things quite well enough to explain its long and otherwise mystifying success through the generations.

## Lydia's Legacy

By far the most enlightening, if unexpected, result of the research program was the discovery that the happy users of the Vegetable Compound might have been enjoying something in the nature of estrogen therapy almost a hundred years before anyone heard the name. Since no known hormonal factors were included in the formula, the newly engaged chemists found themselves considerably puzzled by the "specificity of hormonal therapy ' noted in menopausal studies. They had unsentimentally assumed that the Compound would not be of much value in the treatment of this condition apart, perhaps, from improving sleep, appetite and general health. But since the clinical reports were too consistent to be ignored, they finally felt warranted in investigating the bemusing possibility of estrogenic material somehow concealed in the Compound. Research into the estrogenic properties of plants, a field which had barely begun to be explored, had already revealed that a fairly wide selection of pussywillow, sarsaparilla, wild cherry and yucca, among others contained estrogenic materials, or principles capable of being converted into estrogens by chemical means.

At any rate, the results obtained on bio-assaying extracts of the Compound by the usual methods were so electrifying that the investigators became more than ever severely skeptical, and the extracts were sent, under a code number, to two leading commercial laboratories for independent testing. Both laboratories (one headed by an internationally known figure in the field of endocrinology) confirmed their findings. Having established that the Compound did contain estrogenic material in appreciable quantities, the chemists set to work with renewed impetus and eventually were enabled to determine that two definitely, and possibly three, of its ingredients were mainly responsible.

It was, of course, a far cry from the simple Eclectics of the last century. All that Mrs. Pinkham had noted, or Dr. John King before her, or some anonymous but experimental-minded Indian squaw long before him, was that certain herbs were nature's special gift to women."

*And to us all.*

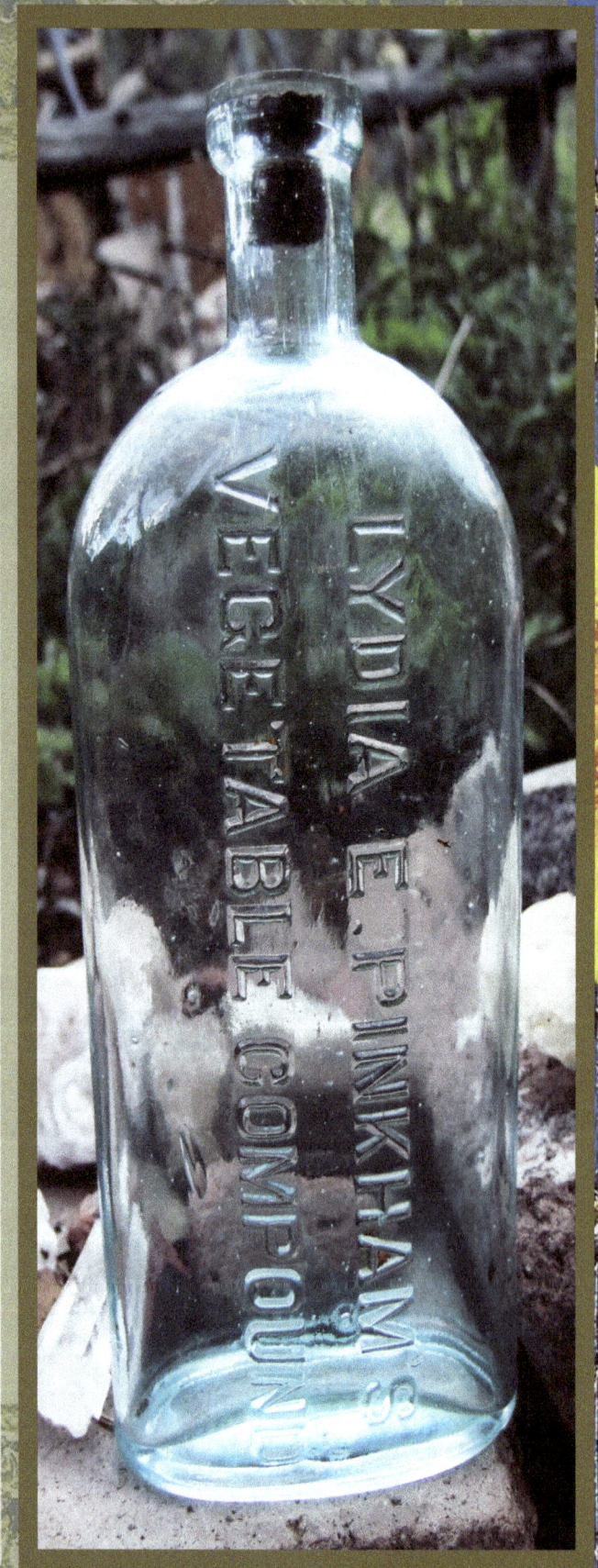

# The Bawdy Ballad of Lydia Pinkham

It wasn't long before Pinkham's Vegetable Compound found its way overseas to Britain, as one of America's first medicinal exports... and not long after that, that it inspired what became one of the most popular Irish drinking songs of all time. It's not recorded what the ostensibly prim and proper Mrs. Pinkham's reaction was, if any, though I like to imagine a secret smile coming over her usually sedate face. You can hear sanitized 1960s versions of the Ballad of Lydia Pinkham on iTunes, performed by both the British band Scaffold and the famed Irish Rovers, and even look up the latest "Club" dance versions. But to enjoy any of the original bawdy lyrics, you'll just have to avail yourselves of the following sampling of authentic lyrics and score, and get to singin' it yourself (a free teeshirt to the first person to belt it at our annual Traditions in Western Herbalism Conference!). Have fun... and remember to drink your vegetables.

Then we'll sing, we'll sing,
We'll sing of Lydia Pinkham,
Savior of the human race.
How she makes, she bottles,
She sells her vegetable compound,
And all the papers print her face.

Widow Brown, she had no children,
Though she loved them very dear,
So she took, she swallowed, she gargled
Some vegetable compound,
And now she has them twice a year
Billy Black lacked hair on his balls,
And his pecker wouldn't peck,
So he took, he swallowed, he gargled
Some vegetable compound,
Now it's as long as a gy-raffe's neck.
Mrs. Jones had rotten kidneys;
Poor old lady couldn't pee,
So she took, she swallowed, she gargled
Some vegetable compound,
And now they pipe her out to sea.
Arthur White had been castrated
And had not a single nut,
So he took, he swallowed, he gargled
Some vegetable compound,
And now they hang all 'round his butt.
Then we'll sing, we'll sing,
We'll sing of Lydia Pinkham,
Savior of the human race.
How she makes, she bottles,
She sells her vegetable compound,
And all the papers print her face.

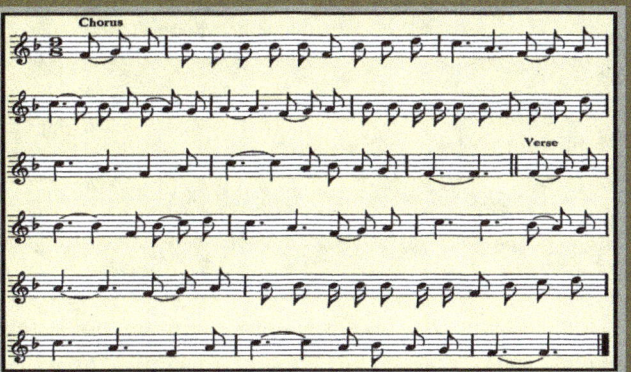

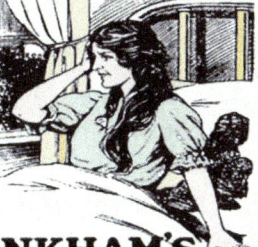

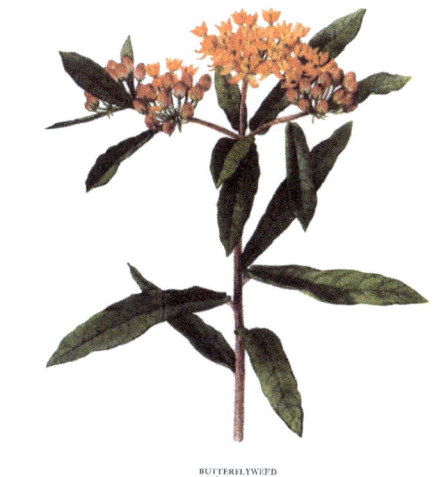

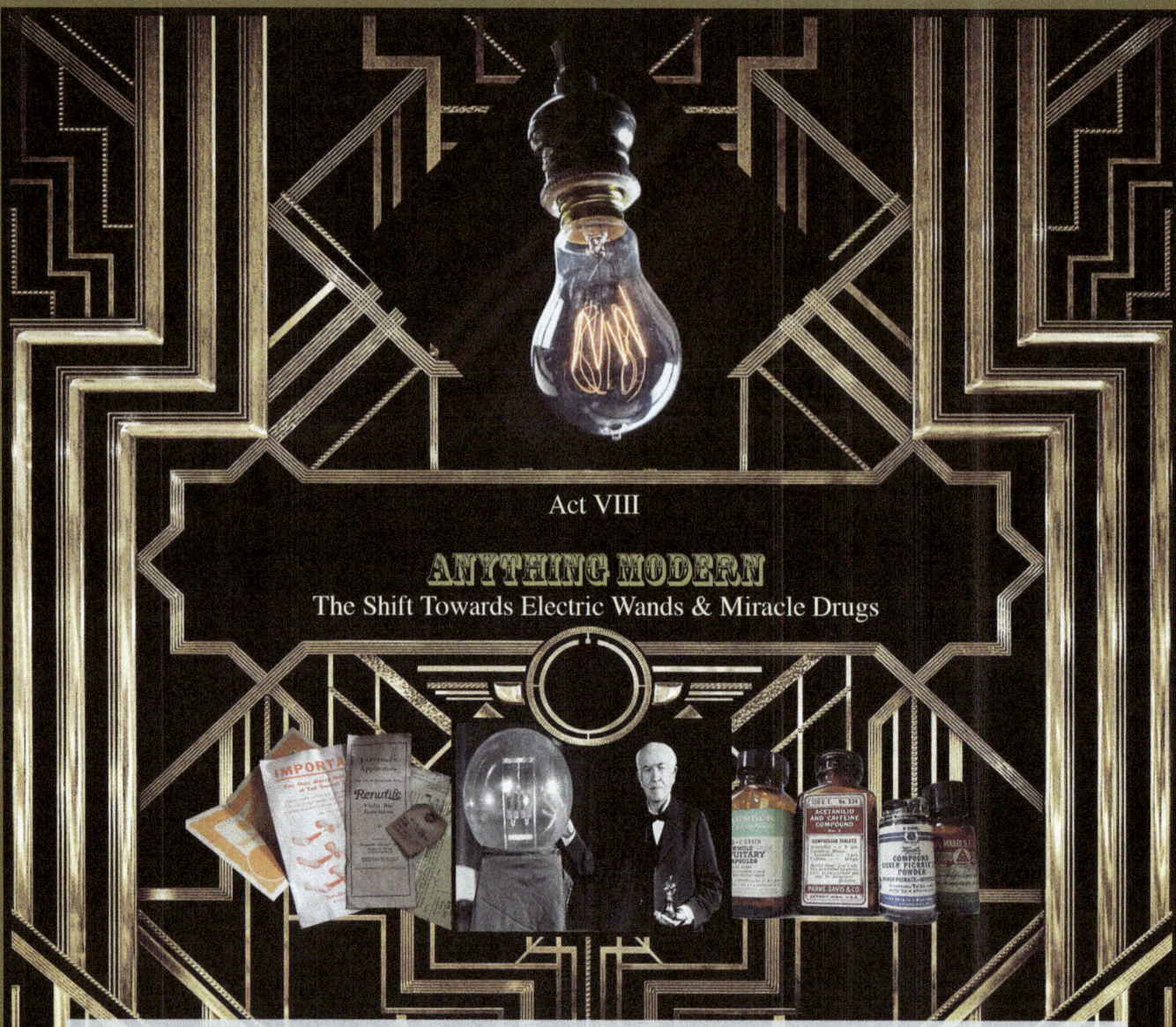

Act VIII

## ANYTHING MODERN
### The Shift Towards Electric Wands & Miracle Drugs

The end of the 1800s marked not only the closing of a Julian century, but a major transition from long revered precepts, traditions and lifestyles. Change had always been a constant, but seldom so great of changes, so quickly and riotously emerging, then so commonly spread, and subsequently so stringently enforced. It could be seen in the dissolution of whole countries and the contorting of alliances, in the rapid evolution of "liberating" fashions, in scientific breakthroughs and technological advancement. Change was in the air, or so said commentators in all fields of human endeavor, entertainment and development. You could see it at the World's Fair, and hear about it on ever more popular radio. The atmosphere, like that newfangled radio, was *electrified*.

There was indeed a new poster child for innovation, with electricity being all that science had promised, and with its own promises being many: new electrically powered machines, capable of either doing or easing the tasks heretofore requiring the long hours and hard labors of humans. First came the electric light, literally and figuratively "illuminating the dark" that people were said to have been so long subject to. Whereas the period of the Enlightenment had been about ideas, now it appeared as a visible reality. Then, pretty soon, it was electric motors and electric powered factories rather than steam; refrigerators instead of genuinely problematic ice boxes. Self-starting automobiles that no longer needed to be hand-cranked. Nothing said "modern new world" like electricity did, a sure sign of the amazing new world to come.

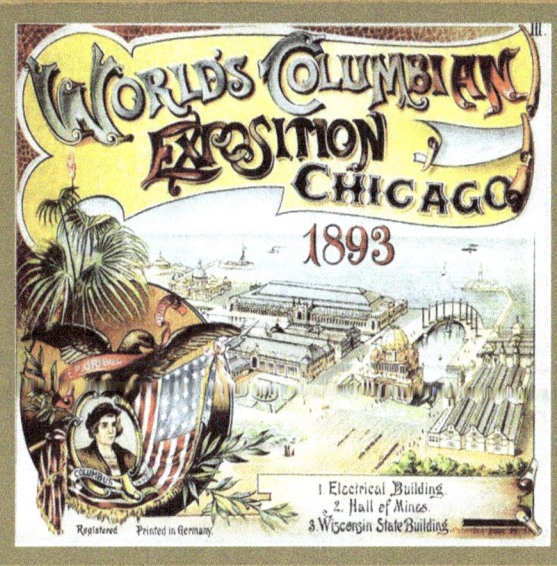
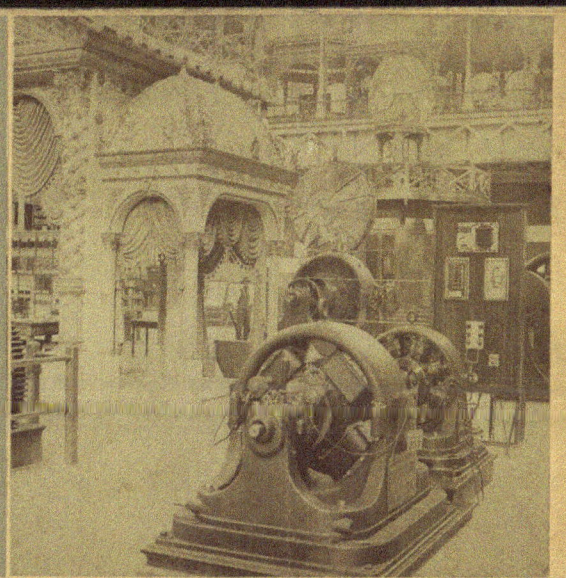

8683. Dynamos and Great Lens, Electric Building, World's Columbian Exposition.

Seeing the "Electric Building" at the 1895 Columbia Exposition helped create a desire for this awesome new power in almost everyone. Within twenty years time, cords would be seen dangling from all manner of new appliances, both frivolous and needed, and so it should be no surprise that it was to electricity that marketers and their ailing customers also looked for the most modern, up-to-date "cures." After all, no "forward thinking person" would possibly do any different.

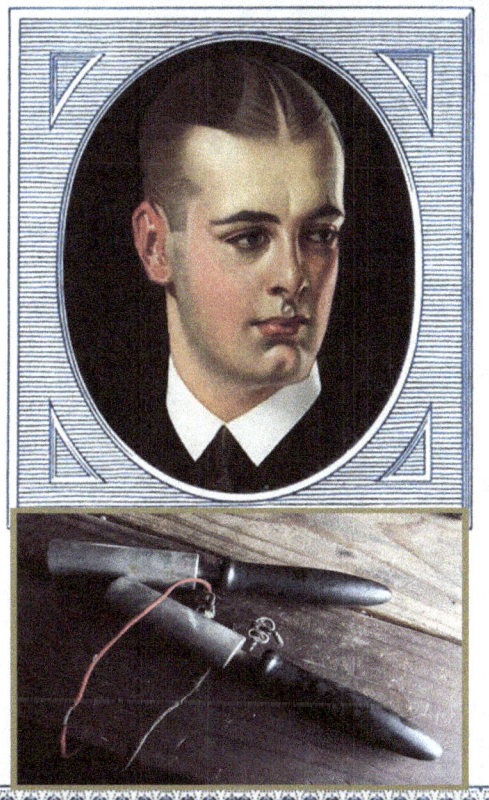

### DR McINTOSH'S GALVANIC AND FARADIC BATTERY.

This celebrated Battery combines both the Galvanic and Faradic, or induced current which can be used separate or in combination.

We claim superiority over all other batteries for the reason that by the improved plan of construction and close connections we gain more quantity and intensity of current. We combine all that is desirable in either a Galvanic or Faradic Battery, a combination never before attained. We furnish it with or without the Faradic coil. It weighs less than any other of the same power. It can be carried without spilling the fluid, thus being the only perfect portable Galvanic Battery made. We will be pleased to send circulars giving full information, price, etc., free, on application.

**McINTOSH GALVANIC BELT AND BATTERY CO.,**

There was no Medicine Show that could "hold a candle" to the brilliant displays of medical technology, including an entirely innefective host of plug-in "Electric Invigorators," "Violet Ray" wands, "Electric Girdles," "Electric Roller," Dr. "Cornflakes" Kellog's "Electric Light Bath," and even several cordless phenomena such as "Electric Magnetic Bathing Fluid" and a so-called "Electric Hairbrush"...
no batteries required!

## THE NEW WAY IN Rheumatism

Rheumatism is very, very painful. Every rheumatic knows that. Rheumatism, under old methods, required very complicated treatment. And every rheumatic knows that.

Doctor Kellogg's leading article in the May GOOD HEALTH shows that medicines are absolutely useless in fighting rheumatism. He shows that the application of heat is the very first step. But it is of vast importance that heat be applied in the most effective way—the Battle Creek way—

### THE ELECTRIC LIGHT BATH

There is no water to heat, no fomentation cloths to get ready, no wet bedding, no chilling of the patient, no irritation of the sensitive skin by hot cloths. Turn a button and the bath is ready. The cost of operation is less than five cents a bath. The results are prompt and permanent, for the Electric Light Bath eliminates the poisons that produce the disease. Used for the treatment of rheumatism in all the great Sanitariums.

**Sent on Appro...**
This Home Bath, just as eff... as our Sanitarium models,... on 30 days FREE TRIAL.... it as you please. Keep i... suits.

Busy men and women find in the cleansing sweat of the Battle Creek Elec... Bath a vital, daily tonic. It brings the buoyancy, life and vigor of perfect... creases efficiency, adds to the joy of living. The Battle Creek Electric Light... practical investment for every home; is in full operation at the mere tur... —gives life long service—costs only 4c a bath.

**Special Introductory Price Offer**— To introduce the ... Elec... Light Bath — for a limited time... are making a special introductory price offer. At moderate cost you can have in you... home the same scientific treatments the greatest Sanitariums use. Write for fre... book of "Home Treatments" and special 30-day introductory offer.

**SANITARIUM EQUIPMENT CO., - Battle Creek, Mich...**

## Physician's Directions for Renulife Treatments
by Noble M. Eberhart M.D., Ph.D., D.C.L.

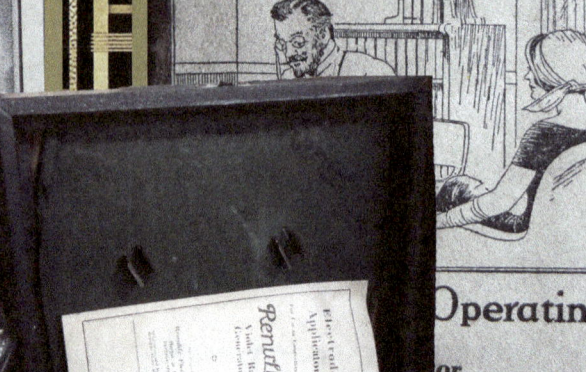

Operating

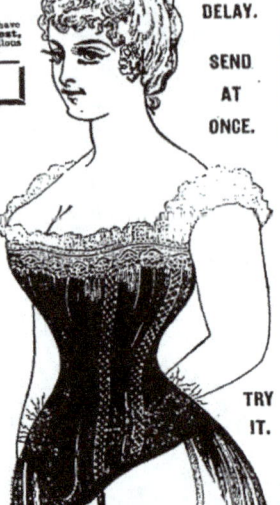

## Ladies in all Stations of Life
# HARNESS' ELECTRIC CORSET.
**BEAUTIFULLY DESIGNED.    SCIENTIFICALLY CONSTRUCTED.    COMFORTABLE TO WEAR.**

**A BOON TO SUFFERERS.**    **5/6**

### HARNESS' ELECTRIC CORSET
...should be worn daily in place of the ordinary one; it will always do good, and never harm. There is no sensation whatever felt in wearing it, while beneficial always and quickly follows. It soon INVIGORATES the entire system, and assists nature in the

**Healthy Development of the Chest.**

Ladies residing in the Country, and those who are unable to call and personally inspect these Corsets, have only to send correct waist measurement with postal orders, and they will obtain, by return of post, **the prettiest, best-fitting Corset** they have ever worn. Its high-class style and beautiful finish, combined with its marvellous health-giving properties, have always won the highest reputation among the leaders of fashion.

**DON'T DELAY. SEND AT ONCE.**

IN appearance they do not differ from the regular corsets, being made of the same material (best quality), in the latest style, and most approved shapes.

**FOR HEALTH, COMFORT, AND ELEGANCE.**

These Beautifully Designed
**CORSETS CURE "WEAK BACK."**

Mrs. FOWLER, Prestwood Road, Heath Town, writes: "I have received great benefit from wearing your Electric Corsets; the pain at the bottom of my back was so bad at times I could not stand, but since wearing your Corsets I feel a new woman."

**"NO WOMAN SHOULD BE WITHOUT ONE!"**

### THE "VERY THING" FOR LADIES.

**BILIOUSNESS.**
Miss LILY, Newport, Mon., writes: "I have obtained great relief from wearing your Electric Corsets. For two or three years I suffered from Biliousness; but since wearing the Corset for three or four months I feel quite well, and have not had an attack."

**INDIGESTION.**
Miss MASON, 3, The Lawn, St. Leonards-on-Sea, writes: "I was suffering from Indigestion and Poorness of Blood; now I feel very much better in health, and have only had one attack of Indigestion since March, and before I was hardly free from pain in the chest."

**5/6 ELECTRIC CORSET**

TRY ONE,... WILL... WEAR... KIND.

**FOR HEALTH, COMFORT, AND ELEGANCE.**

...perfectly designed Corset the most awkward figure becomes graceful and elegant, the internal organs are speedily strengthened, and the entire system is invigorated.

**...ALLY DESIGNED CORSETS FOR CHILDREN.**
...ALLY DESIGNED ELECTRIC CORSET is the Acme of Perfection for children of all ages. It is scientifically ... recommended. It gives perfect support, prevents stooping, and is an effectual guard against chills...

**TRY IT.**

...D AT ONCE Postal Order or Cheque for one of these beautiful Corsets.
PRICE ONLY 5s. 6d., POST FREE.

**...MEDICAL BATTERY CO., LTD.,**
**...OXFORD ST. LONDON. W.**

**BONNORE'S CURES** — PARALYSIS, NERVOSIS, MEASLES, FEMALE COMPLAINTS, RHEUMATISM, CHRONIC ABSCESS, MERCURIAL ERUPTIONS, CHOLERA, EPILEPSY, SCARLET FEVER, NEURALGIA
**ELECTRO MAGNETIC BATHING FLUID.**

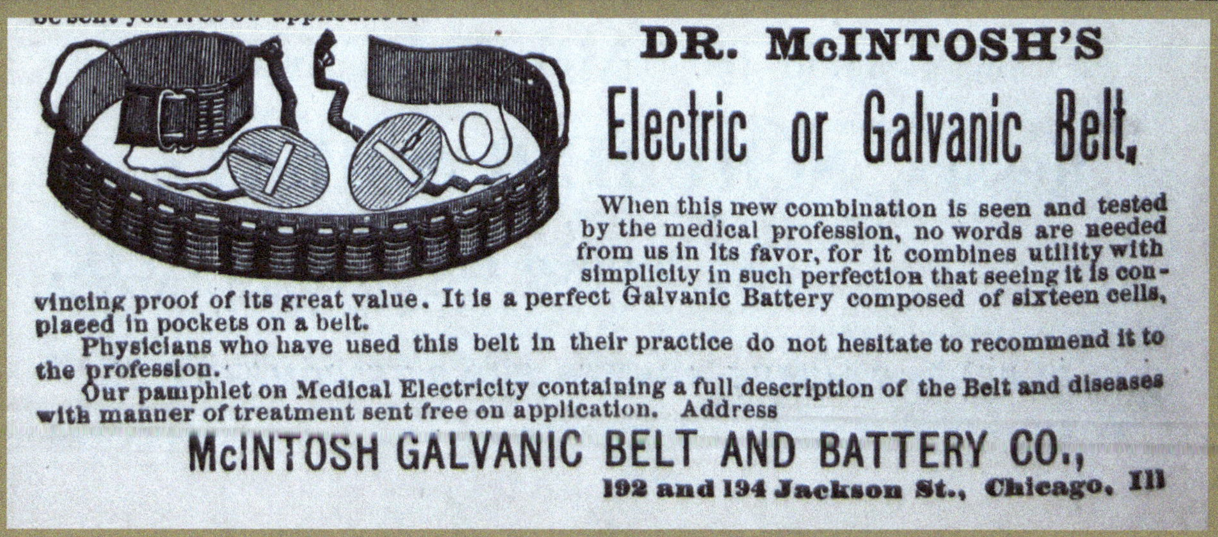

DR. McINTOSH'S
Electric or Galvanic Belt.
When this new combination is seen and tested by the medical profession, no words are needed from us in its favor, for it combines utility with simplicity in such perfection that seeing it is convincing proof of its great value. It is a perfect Galvanic Battery composed of sixteen cells, placed in pockets on a belt.
Physicians who have used this belt in their practice do not hesitate to recommend it to the profession.
Our pamphlet on Medical Electricity containing a full description of the Belt and diseases with manner of treatment sent free on application. Address
McINTOSH GALVANIC BELT AND BATTERY CO.,
192 and 194 Jackson St., Chicago, Ill

ELECTRIC

Directions for using the New No. 4 D.D. Home Medical Apparatus
WITH MESCO DRY CELL BATTERY.

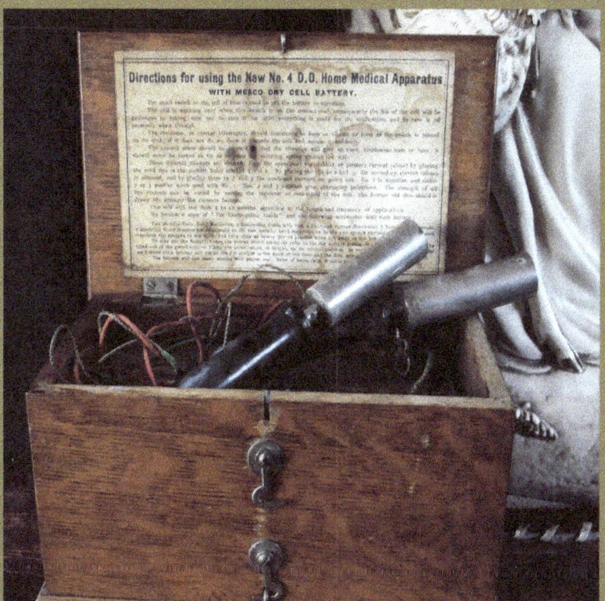

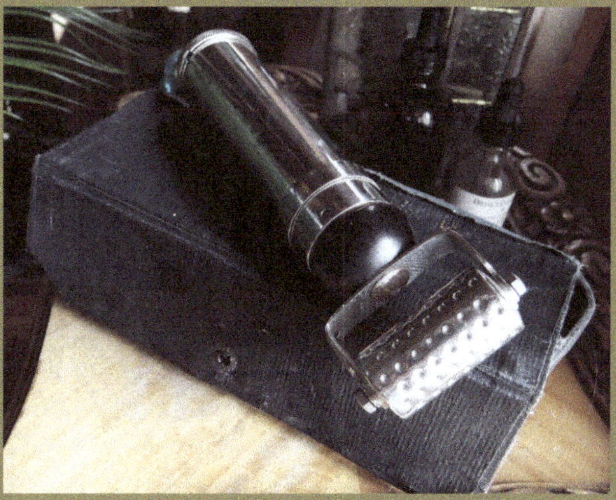

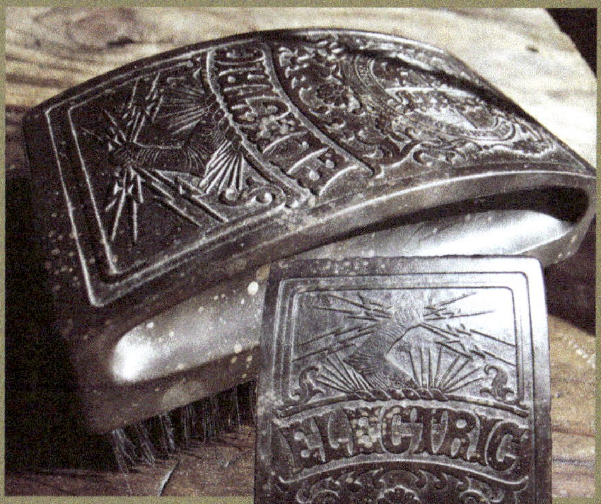

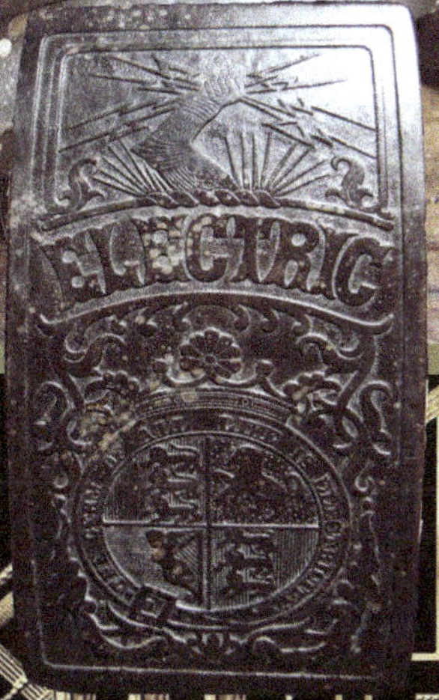

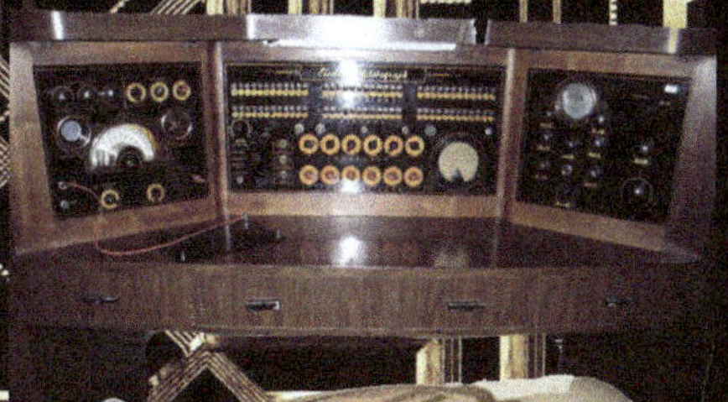

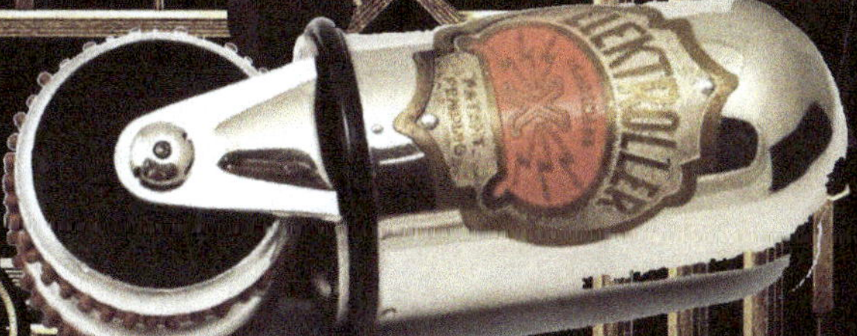

Needless to say, modern women found much more creative uses for their Vitapulsers... than tickling their chins...

# How to use The *Vitapulser*

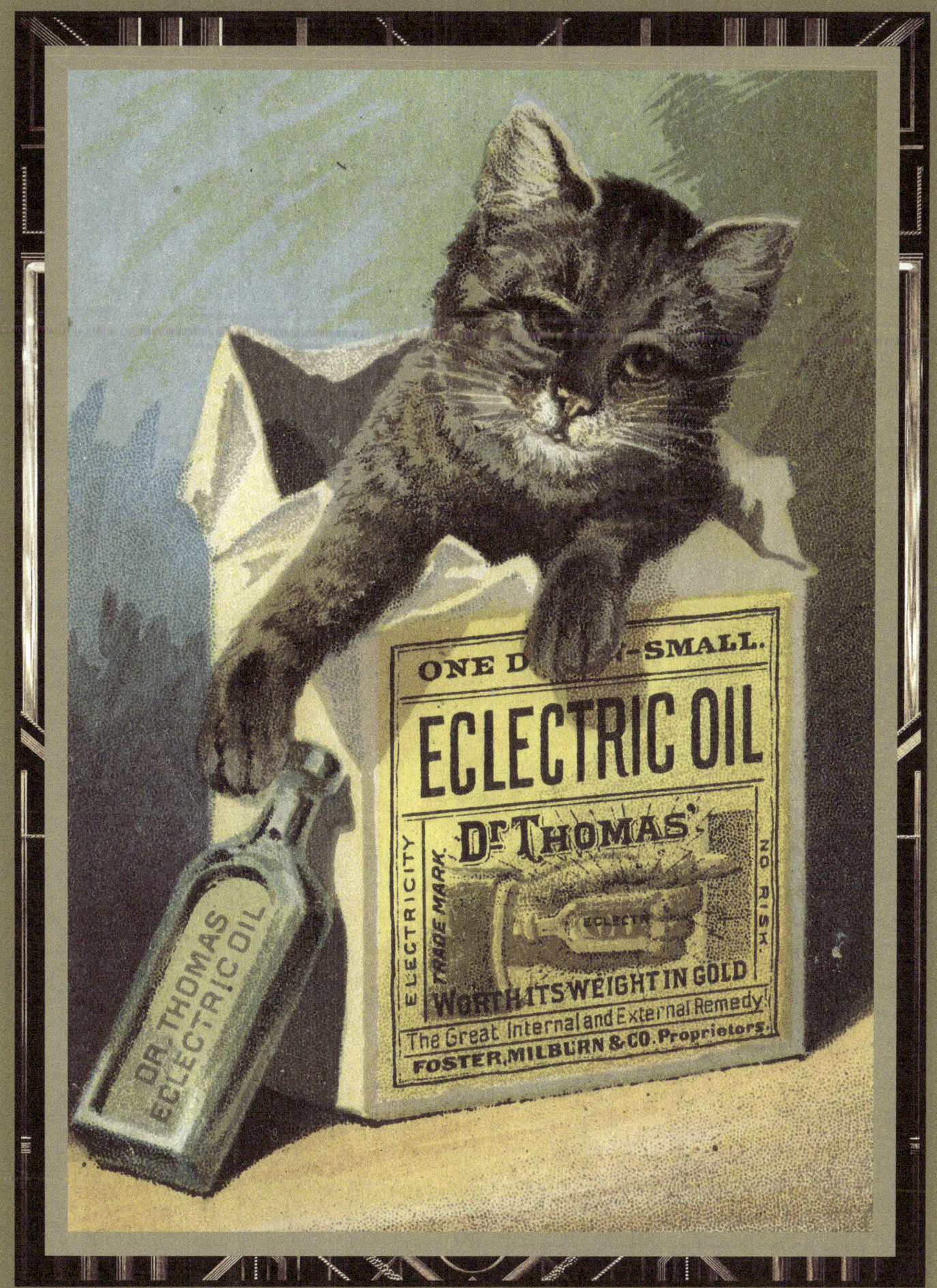

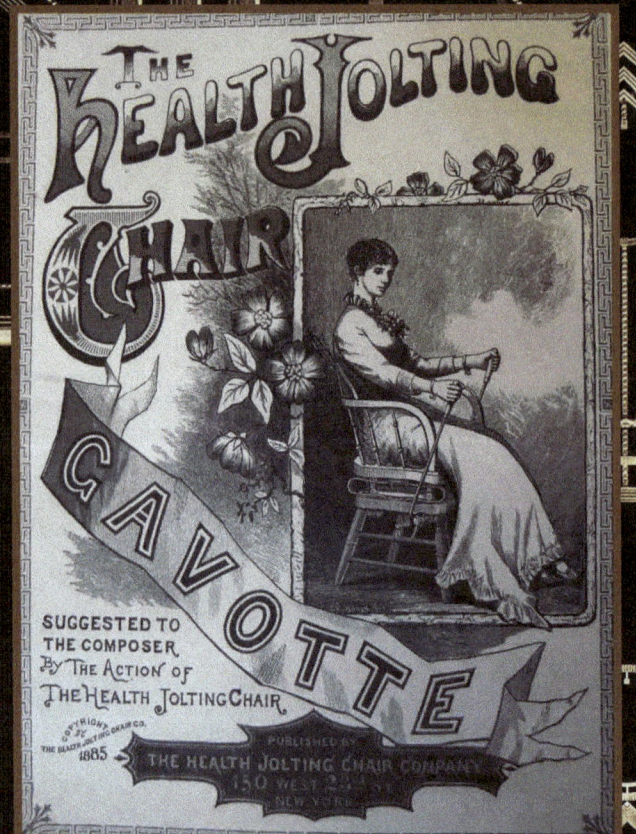

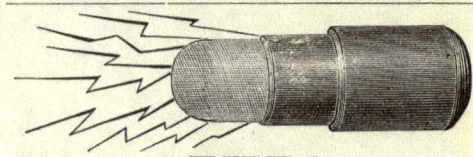

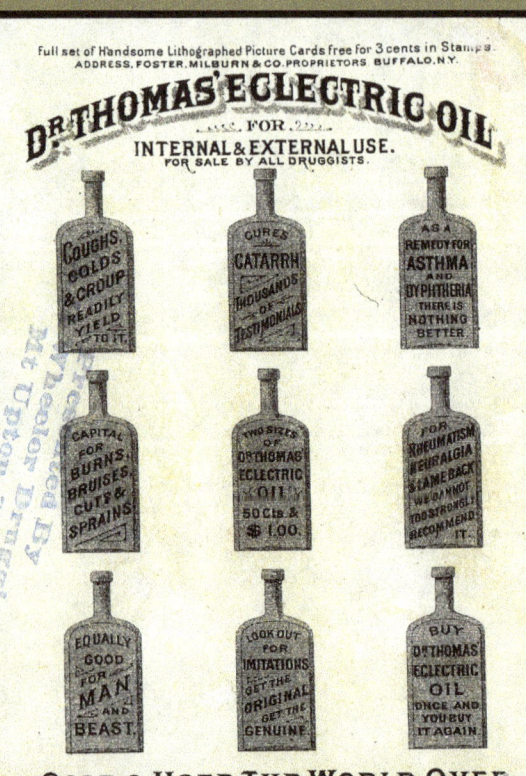

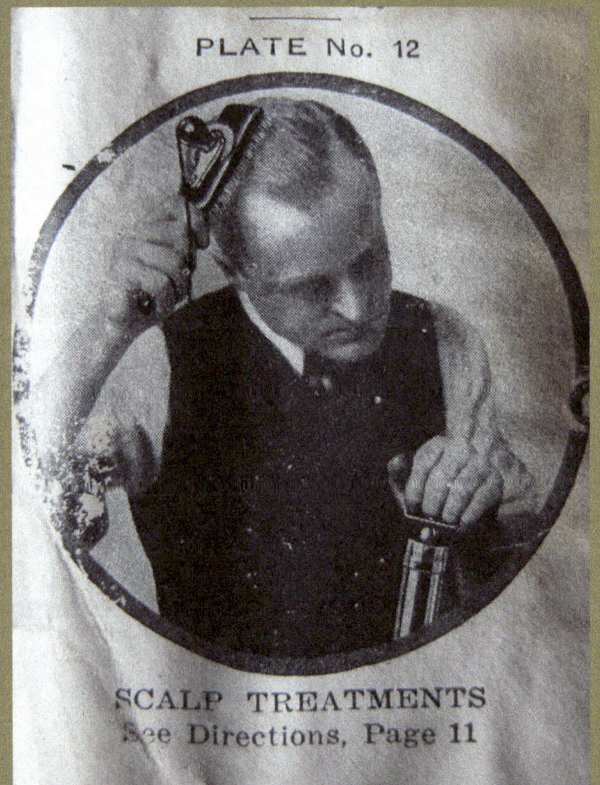

Not all of the modern medical devices that folks flocked to were "electrified," of course, nor were designed for application to one's bottom.... but judging by some of the following, it is a darn good thing.

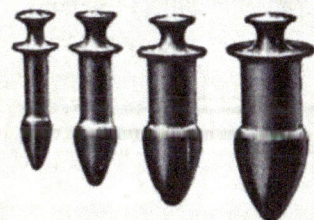

### IN PILES AND CONSTIPATION

The best results may be obtained by the use of ... YOUNG'S self-retaining ...

### RECTAL DILATORS

They are made of hard rubber and come in sets of four sizes. May be used by any intelligent person. Their use accomplishes for the invalid just what nature does daily for the healthy individual. If you will prescribe a set of these dilators in some of your obstinate cases of Chronic Constipation you will find them necessary in every case of this kind. Price to the profession, $2.50 per set. Sold by leading instrument houses and

**F. E. YOUNG & CO.,**
46 Michigan Avenue, - CHICAGO

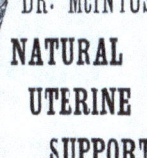

### McINTOSH GALVANIC BELT AND BATTERY CO.,
Nos. 192 and 194 Jackson St., Chicago, Ill.

### DR. McINTOSH'S NATURAL UTERINE SUPPORTER

No instrument has ever been placed before the medical profession which has given such universal satisfaction. The combination is such that the Physician is able to meet every indication of Uterine Displacements. Falling Womb, Anti-version, Retroversion and Flexions are overcome by this instrument, where others fail; this is proven by the fact that since its introduction to the Profession it has come into more general use than all other instruments combined.

The Abdominal Supporter is a broad morocco leather belt with elastic straps to buckle around the hips, with concave front, so shaped as to hold up the abdomen. The Uterine Support is a cup and stem made of highly-polished hard rubber very light and durable, shaped to fit the neck of the womb, with openings for the secretions to pass out; as shown by the cuts. Cups are made with extended lips to correct flexions and versions of the womb.

The instrument is very comfortable to the patient, can be removed or replaced by her at will, can be worn by her at all times, will not interfere with nature's necessities, will not corrode, and is lighter than metal. It will answer for all cases of Anteversion, Retroversions, or any Flexions of the Womb and is used by the leading Physicians with never-failing success even in the worst cases.

Price to Physicians, $6.00; to Patients, $10. ... our risk, on receipt of price, or by Express, C. O. D., with the ... money added. ... sale and popularity of our instrument, various and ... ous parties. In order to get the genuine, it is best to

**... AL UTERINE SUPPORTER CO.,**
... EET, CHICAGO, ILL.

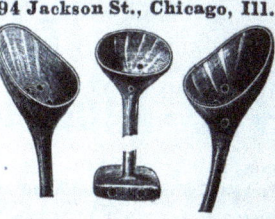

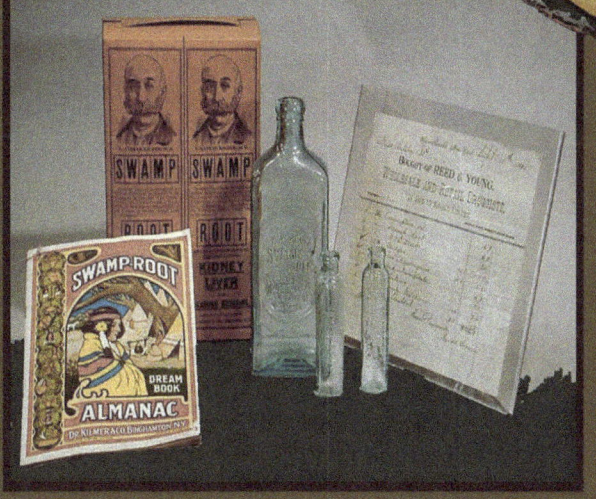

Products like the one above, mark the major transition point between the two paradigms, being mass produced and commercially packaged like the drugs that would follow, and yet still being marketed at a time when an association with "Indians" and "Swamps" could translate into brisk sales.

While there were certainly cases of people suffering shocks from using faulty electrical "cures," most of these devices proved to be as harmless as they were fruitless. Considerably more dangerous have been chemicals marketed to folks for the past hundreds of years, and the synthesized pharmaceutical drugs that all "modern thinking" people seemed to be switching to by the 20th Century. This shift in the health paradigm went hand in hand with the migration of the American population from farms, ranches, and small towns, to the largest cities where economic opportunities and a genteel lifestyle awaited them. With each generation away from the land, nature apparently began to seem more alien, less relevant, less understandable, and increasingly foreboding. Plants were for outside in the garden or yard now, while bottled medicines were for indoors, the places where people were beginning to spend most of their mortal days.

Apothecaries featured fresh whole herbs grown or gathered locally, as well as custom blended medicines in various forms, created by a knowledgable plant healer. A customer could expect helpful advice, along with a potential remedy with minimal likelihood of it causing any problems, and almost no chance of it resulting in a death. In a period of less than 50 years, nearly all American apothecaries were supplanted by the "modern drug store," selling packaged medicines made by distant corporations, and meting out measured doses of prescribed chemicals. The druggist would no longer be available for advice, legally bound to leave all recommendations to a licensed physician whether the customer could afford that service or not. This was arguably a good idea, since a mistake in diagnosis, pharmaceutical medicine or dosage could now easily damage or kill a person.

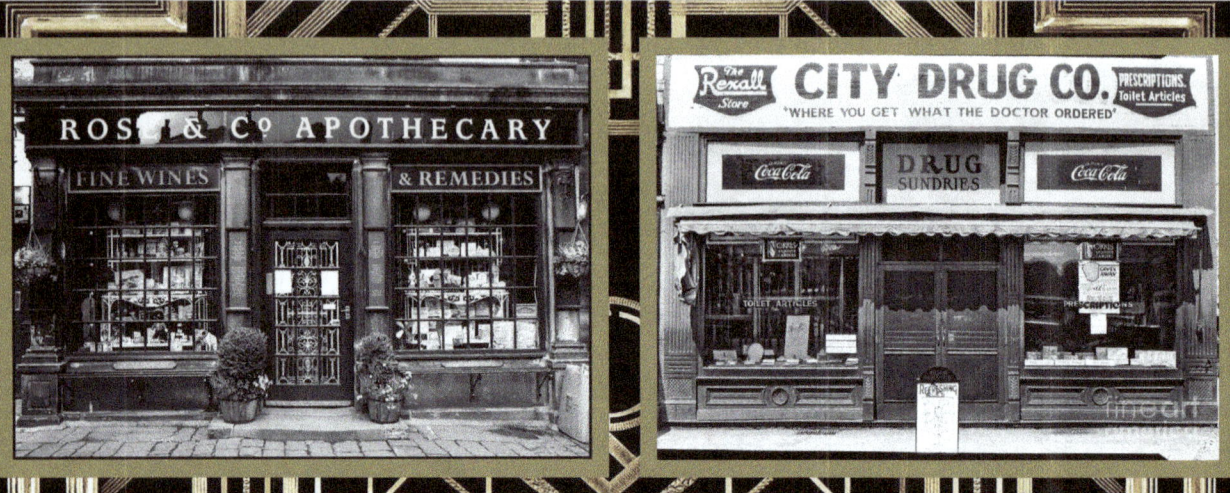

The change could be seen not only in the disappearance of the town apothecary and community health care providers, but also in the absence of jars of whole herbs on the shelves of America's stores. In their stead, a buyer could find all manner of processed medicines, first with labels bragging about the plants they were derived from, then later avoiding any such mention. Products like Hunt's Remedy not only didn't say a word about herbs, but also exemplified the new attitude of battling with illness and death. The traditional herbalist/healer's approach of boosting the body's own healing, and seeking balance within the bodily and larger natural ecosystems, gave way in advertising as well as in the doctor's office to a language of "killing germs" and "waging war" against illness. The folk healer's emphasis on preventive health care through nutrition and tonics was set aside and largely forgotten. It no longer seemed to matter so much how one ate, how much exercise they got, or what other healthy precautions might be taken, since modern medicine could be expected to "fix" whatever damage might be done.

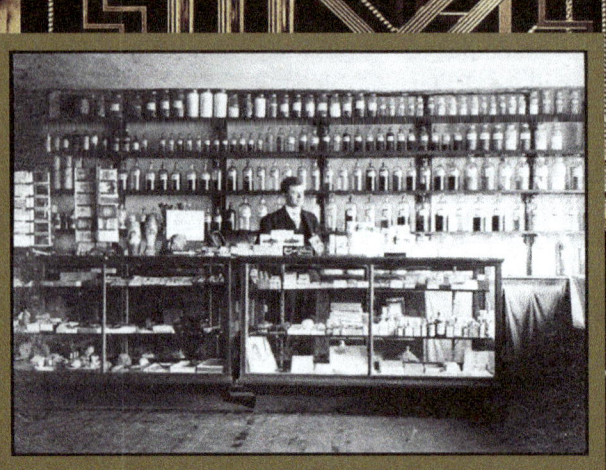
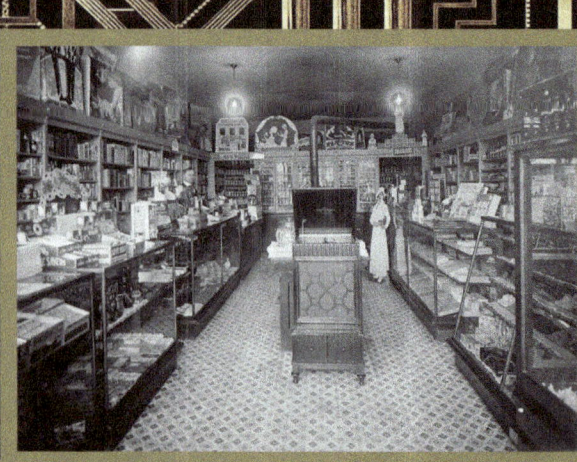

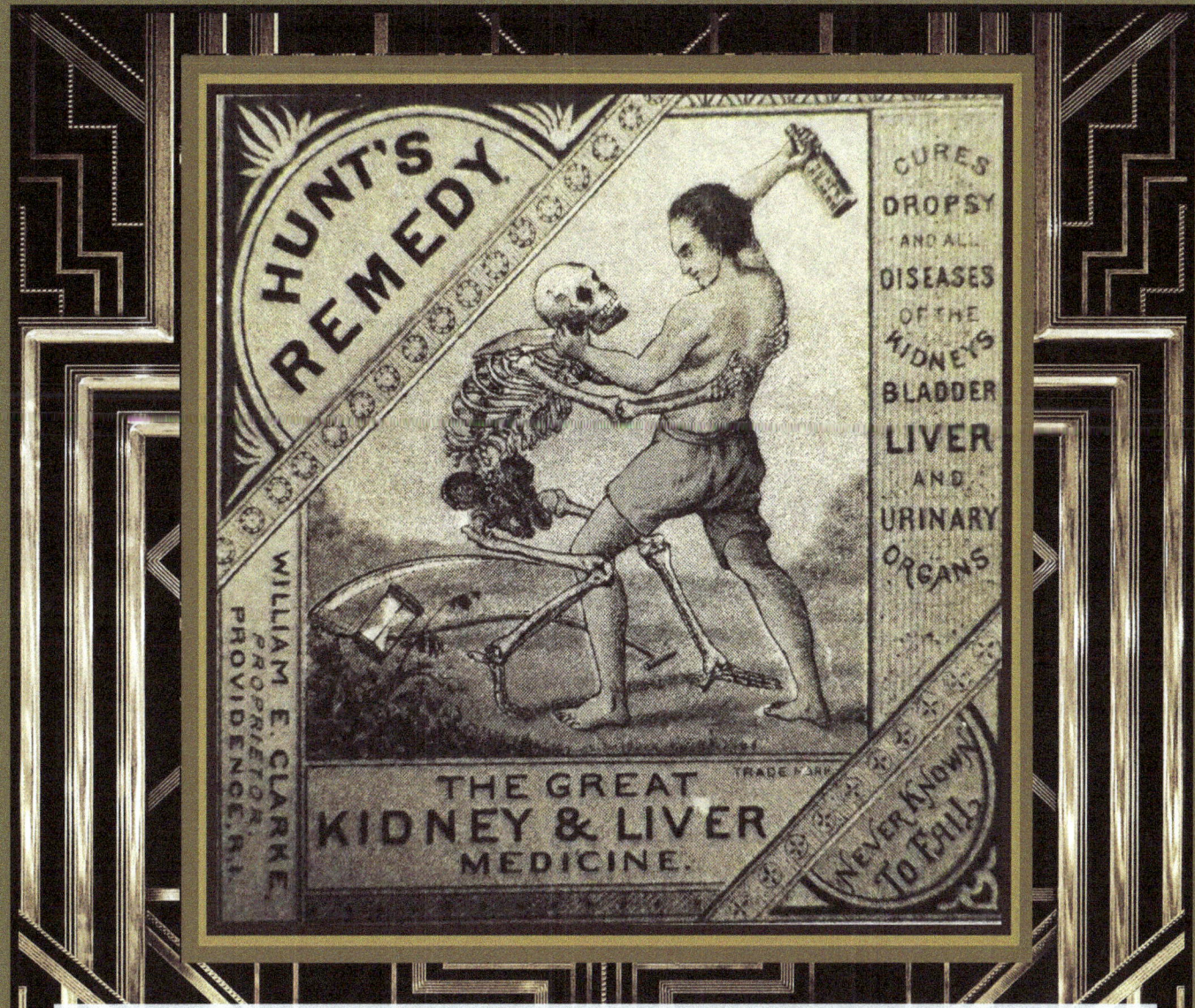

From 1900 to 2000, herbs were more and more often dismissed in American households for being less powerful than the new wonder drugs, as well as for being messier, and more time consuming. Medicines like tinctures, decoctions and teas made from whole plants lacked the appeal of the newly synthesized chemicals in their tidy and handy little capsules. Nature is crude, imperfect, and inconvenient, people said, while modern science and technology promised to quickly and certainly usher humanity into a preprogrammed future of comfort, longevity, and the virtual abolition of disease.

Throughout, there was resistance from a natural healing counterculture, not only the ostracized and vilified practitioners in danger of losing their livelihood to new regulations, but also from nonprofessionals: from the Amish and Native Americans; from rural families with generations of following an Appalachian, Southwestern/Hispanic or other natural healing tradition; from folks who couldn't afford store-bought goods even if they preferred them, as well as from those with plenty of money but a strong commitment to natural healing; not just from show operators or their herbal medicine producers, but also from those who made their small batches of medicines atop kitchen tables for free use by anyone living in the neighborhood, and who had never even beheld the pitchmen and plant healers of the traveling Medicine Shows.

Frightening to all of these, were not only society's shift in interest, buying trends and attitudes, but what they also knew to be impending modern legislation, favoring big business, and making it ever harder for either herbalism or the shows to survive.

# Act IX
## DENIGRATION & LEGISLATION

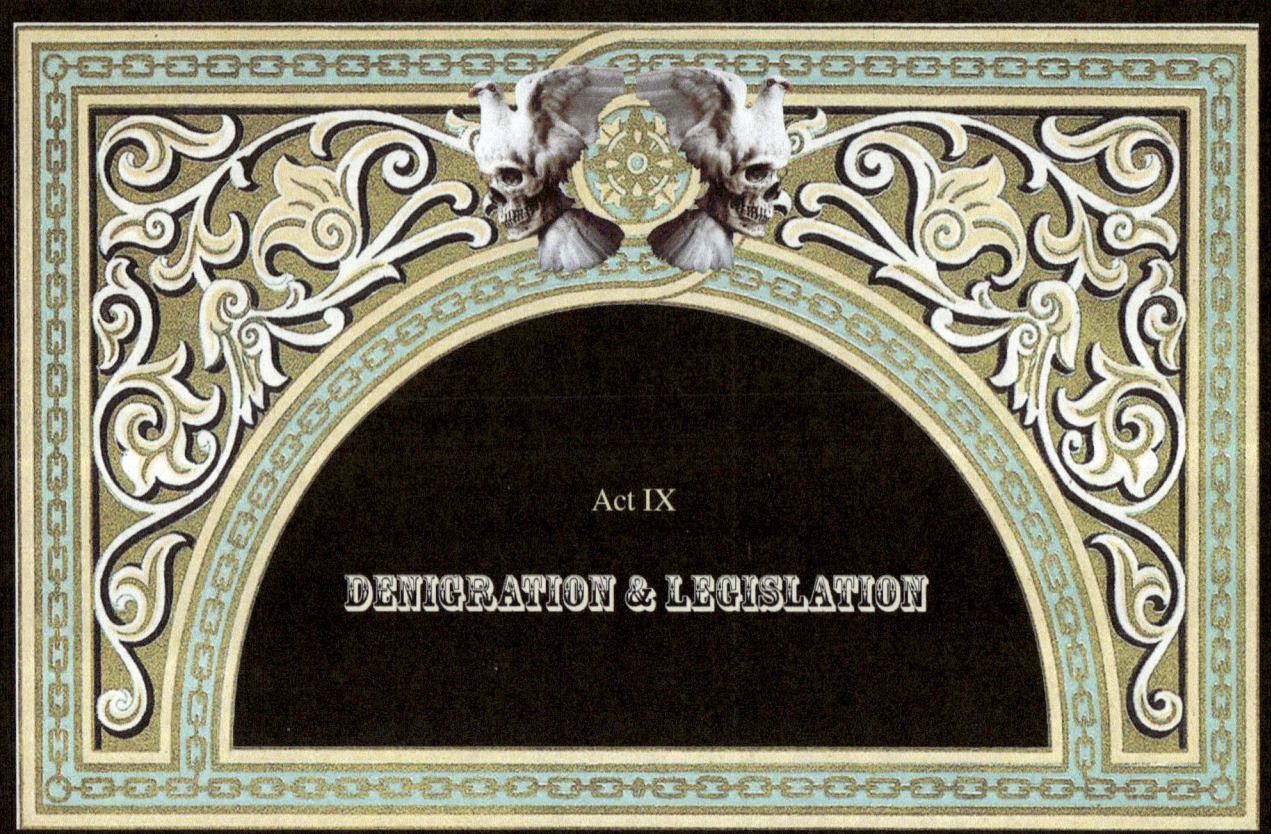

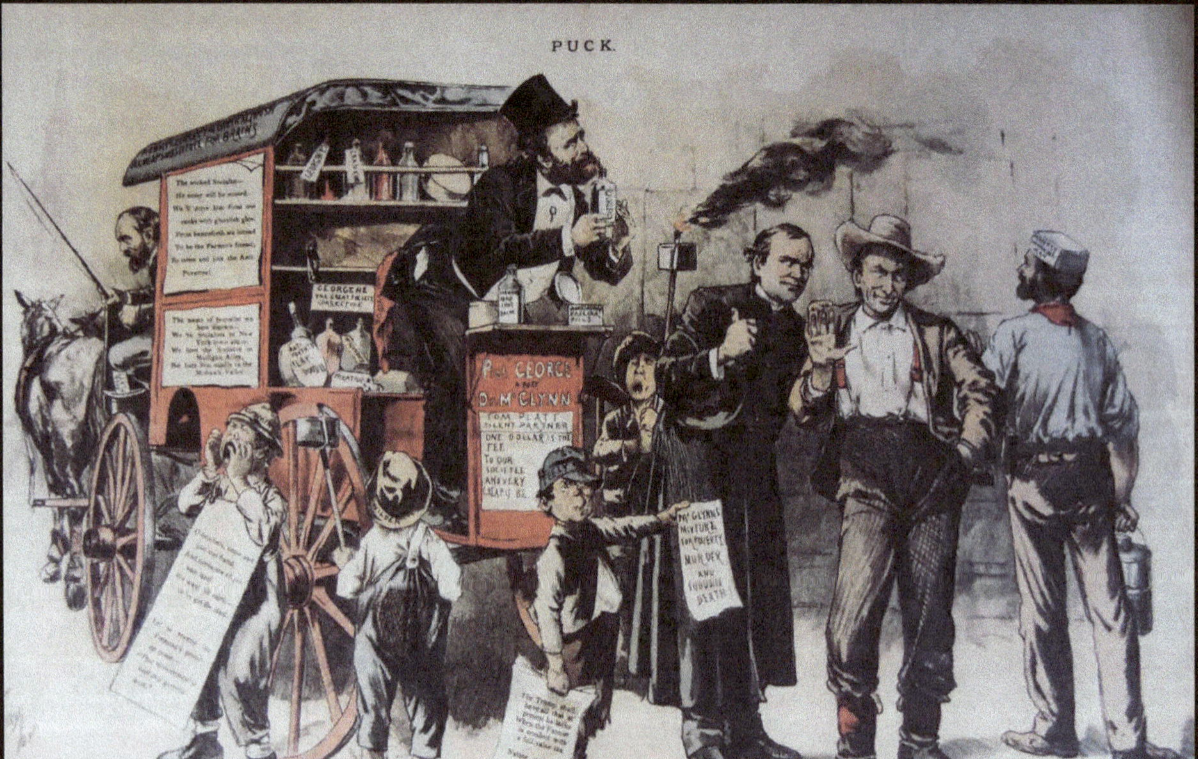

THE GREAT QUACKERY "COMBINE" ON ITS TRAVELS.

The Traveling Medicine Shows suffered attacks from their very inception. The primary complainants, however, were almost never the locals who plopped down their hard earned money for a bottle of "Doc Regent's Lifeforce Tonic," but rather, from the rapidly expanding industrial manufacturers and professional medical organizations who labeled all non-vetted practitioners as "quacks" and all non-proprietary treatments as "bunk." As early as 1757, the royal colonist William Smith wrote that "Quacks abound like Locusts in Egypt and too may have recommended themselves to full Practice and profitable Subsistence." Legislation regulating "mountebank" medicine sellers was passed by New Jersey and Connecticut lawmakers in 1772 and 1773, a freedom restricting move predating the U.S. Declaration of Independence by a full three years.

Medicine Shows continued to gain in popularity between 1776 and the 1850s, in spite of the new laws and prejudices against them. And with Andrew Jackson's ascent to the United States presidency, a philosophy of egalitarianism and emphasis on the rights of the common man had at least temporary support from the top. Licensing laws for physicians were suspended, and boards of approval no longer were allowed to supplant the ages old systems of patient experience and practitioner reputation.

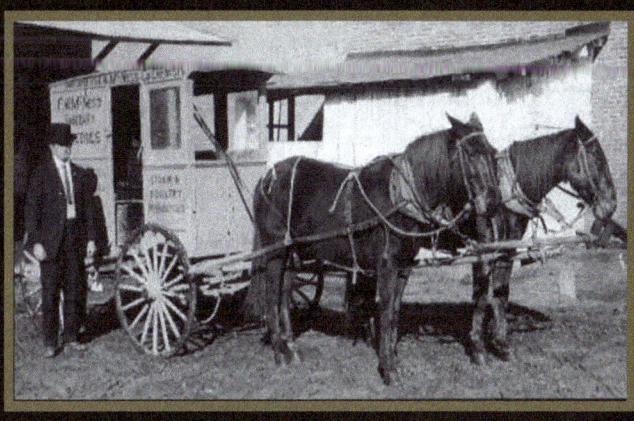

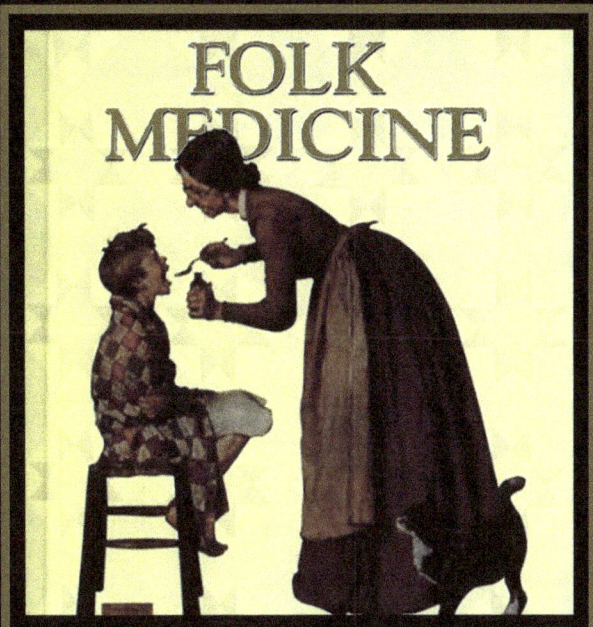

As a result, the ranks of doctors swelled to include large numbers of both men and women practitioners, with one effect being a precipitous drop in the prices that physicians could demand for their services. It was this blow to the heretofore exorbitant rates of the "professionals" that triggered the intense enmity and concerted retaliation of their organizations and agencies, resulting in these organization's eventual success at reinstating licensing requirements, membership and privileges... and a prompt return to the characteristically high fees of their once again increasingly elitist ranks. Previously there were unlicensed health care provders who learned through apprenticeship and experience, some of whom were excellent, and some not so. Now only the licensed could practice, some doing it well, and likewise, some not so well.

Simultaneously, unscrupulous companies were taking advantage of the absence of restrictions to include a host of sometimes harmful chemicals in their "health" products, as well as introducing noxious ingredients such as borax as standard food preservatives. Often it was the most impoverished strata of society that suffered the most, being the people most likely to seek cures off the shelves rather than getting a trained assessment and treatment. Tales of users getting ill or dying inspired a host of social activists (referred to as "muckrakers") to actively lobby for laws on behalf of public health, greatly influencing public policy by publishing articles with their mission to "expose the evils of nostrums and false doctors."

One such muckraker, Samuel Hopkins Adams, wrote a highly influential essay "The Great American Fraud" for Collier's Weekly in 1905, pointing to the dangers of such nasty hidden ingredients as "acetanilid," and "antikamnia" commonly found in headache powders, including the brands Orangeine and the best-selling BromoSeltzer.

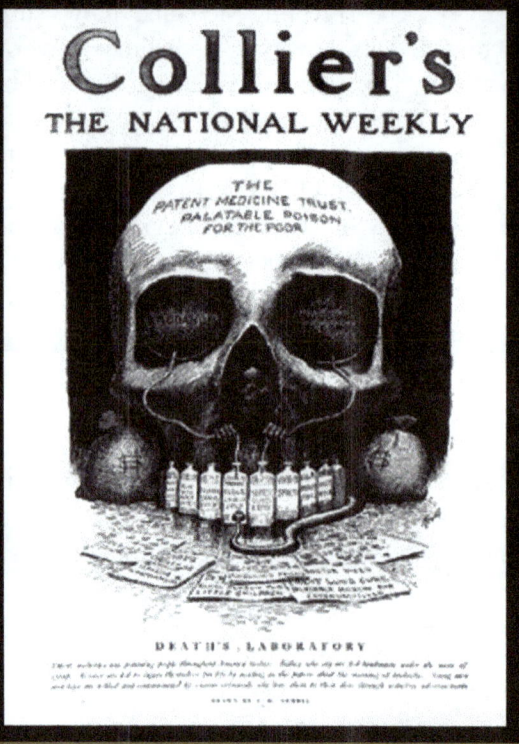

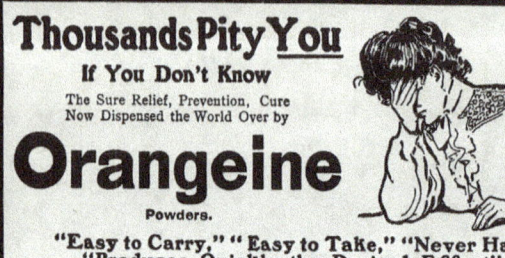

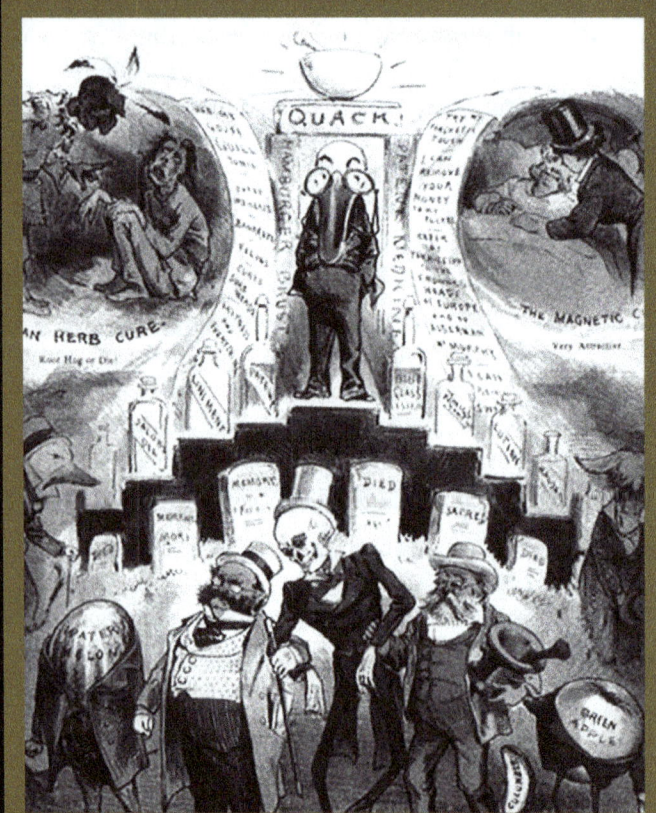

"Gullible America, he wrote, "will spend this year millions of dollars in the purchase of patent medicines. In consideration of this sum it will swallow huge quantities of alcohol, an appalling amount of opiates and narcotics, a wide assortment of varied drugs ranging from powerful and dangerous heart depressants to insidious liver stimulants; and, in excess of all other ingredients, undiluted fraud. For fraud, exploited by the skilfulest of advertising bunco men, is the basis of the trade. Should the newspapers, the magazines and the medical journals refuse their pages to this class of advertisement, the nation would be the richer not only in lives and money, but in drunkards and drug-fiends saved." There can be little doubt that Adams' motivations were based in a genuine desire to help protect the well being of innocent consumers, but he himself recognized the ways in which such legislation would impact the honest makers of healthful plant medicines. "Don't make the mistake of lumping all propriety medicines in one indiscriminate denunciation,'he warned. If a side effect of regulating manufacturing was to put many herbal sellers out of business, he considered it worth it.

Sadly, research has shown that unlike Adams, the majority of those writers and speakers opposing the Medicine Shows were in actuality hired or otherwise funded by professional physician's organizations and/or a coalition of the chemical and drugs industries. Whether their particular assertions were true or unfounded, the fact that they received support or even instruction from the industry impacts their credibility and puts their ethics into question. The sum total of these written attacks, however, did much to propel public opinion, which in turn commanded the attention of lawmakers.

Perhaps no one was more influential than the director of the U.S. Bureau of Chemistry, the controversial Harvey W. Wiley. Wiley's determined investigations into food additives proved a major factor in the passage in 1906 of The Pure Food and Drug Act, first mandating that medicine makers include an accurate list of ingredients on their bottles. Beyond lamenting the cost of printed labels, there were few other objections heard from the herbalists, "root doctors" and "granny-wives" that rural folks and the poorer classes depended upon for their physical well-being. Subsequent legislation, unfortunately, resulted not only in increased consumer protection but also the de facto approval and promotion of chemicals and isolates over plant parts and products, and the ascendancy of medicinal mega-producers over regional mom-and-pop providers – an arc we traced in our look at the "modernization" of the Lydia Pinkham company. As mandated, ingredients would indeed be listed forthwith on food and medicine labels, but note that they would no longer be seen in advertisements. Unlike with wholesome-sounding ingredients such as "celery," "ginseng," "mint" or "wild rose," few consumers would be able to recognize the approved chemicals' names, nor would they likely find such additives increased their desire to buy.

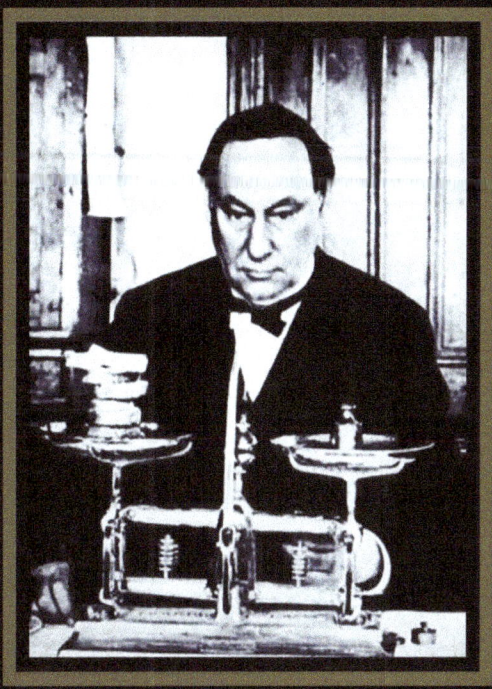

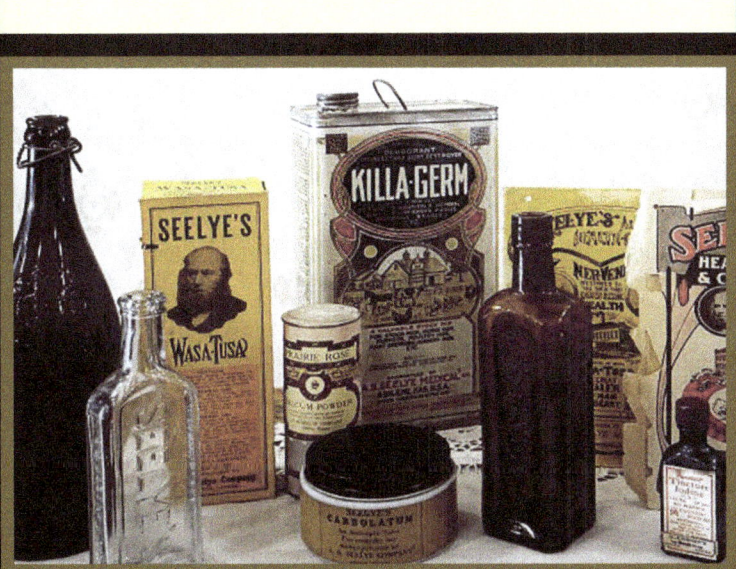

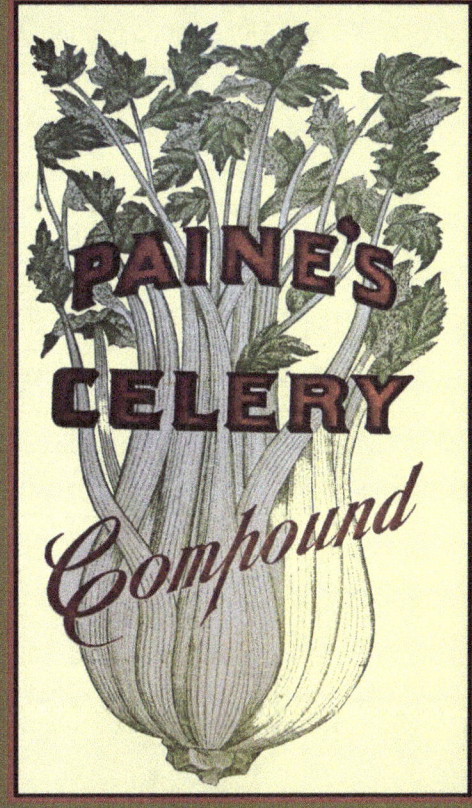

Then, in the 1930s, comes the formation of the Food and Drug Administration (FDA) and Federal Trade Commission (FTC) with complex regulations favoring corporate producers over smalltime businesses. An all out public relations attack was orchestrated at this time by a lamentable alliance of the A.M.A. (American Medical Association) and the APA (American Pharmaceutical Association), together bankrolling, lobbying for, and ultimately pushing through the passage of the Food, Drug and Cosmetic Act of 1938. In earlier bills, businesses were reprimanded for putting possibly harmful chemicals into their products without listing what they were, but beginning in '38, the laws would help ensure that the very largest producers of (still possibly harmful) chemicals would have the official approval and business advantages they needed to effectively corner the market.

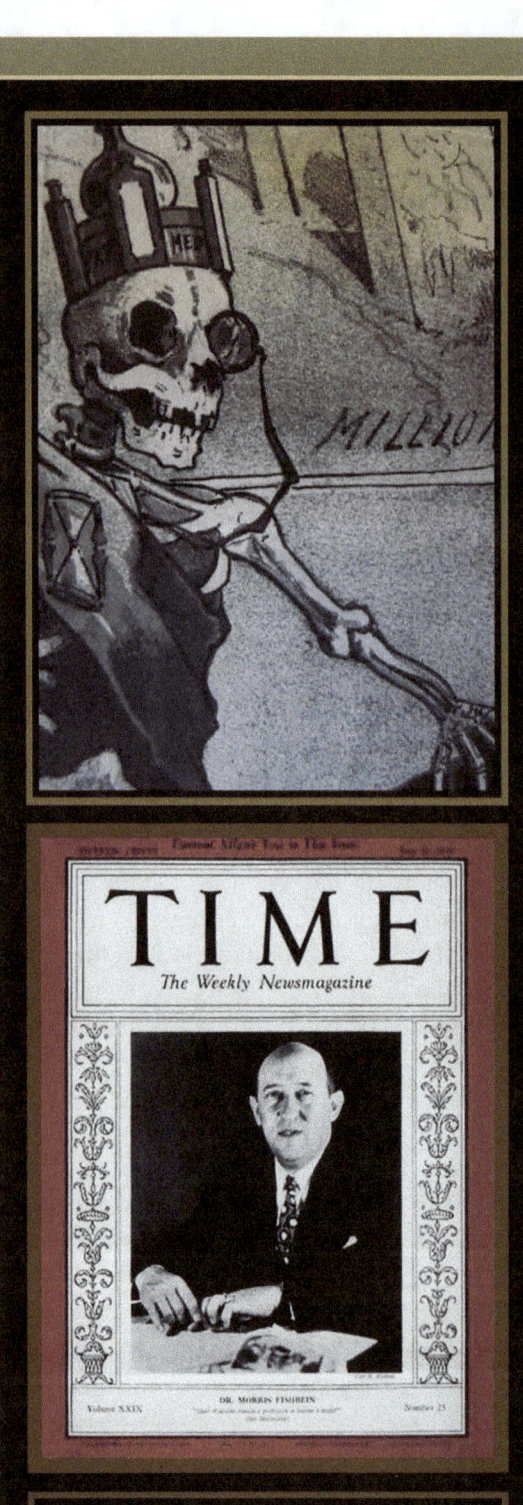

Remarkably, it was also in 1938 that the A.M.A. and its editor of the Journal of The American Medical Association, "Dr." Morris Fishbein, were indicted for violating the provisions of the Sherman Anti-Trust Act, over the AMA's monopoly on professional accreditation. In subsequent testimony, Fishbein was forced to admit that he wasn't even a doctor and had never treated a patient in his life, an ironic fact given that he was kept on as the Medical Association's editor until 1950 primarily on the merits of his constant attacks on all manner of health practitioners not belonging to the A.M.A.! Along with any public service that the 1938 F.D.A. act may have provided, it also imposed a hardship on and helped to ostracize and marginalize herbalism, helping sound the death knell for the traveling Medicine Show, and within another 20 years had turned general public opinion against herbs and natural healing in all but the most remote settlements. Not until the 1960s would there again be a movement fighting for the acceptance of plant medicine efficacy and the legitimization of herbal practice.

Today, there are a huge amount of websites, journals and other publications by industry shills and catty licensed physicians that continue to be dedicated to the "exposing of quacks." I am afraid Fishbein would be proud. Under their definitions of "quackery," we often find a list of "errant and misleading" practices that includes not just questionable treatments like ionic cleansing, colloidal silver and glucosomine supplements, but also such tried and respected fields as herbalism, traditional Chinese medicine, acupuncture, aromatherapy, holistic dentistry, osteopathy, chiropractic practice, and complimentary medicine!

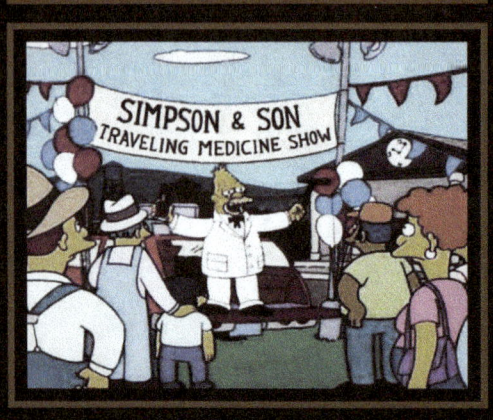

# RYMAN'S RHEUMATIC NEPENTHE

FOR

Sprains, Bruises, Sweeny, Burns, Quinsy, Mumps, Pains of the Back and Limbs.

FOR SALE HERE.

## Henry George's SYSTEM REGULATOR

Alcohol not over 14%
Rhubarb, Cascara and Phenalphthalein
An EFFECTIVE COMPOUND for the relief of CONSTIPATION, BILIOUSNESS and HEADACHES due to constipation.

DOSE—Adults, teaspoonful in a little water after meals 3 times a day as a laxative for sick headache and sick stomach. As a purgative or cathartic, ½ to 1 tablespoonful night and morning.
Children, 8 to 12 years half quantity
Laxatives should not be used when symptoms of appendicitis are present

SHAKE WELL BEFORE USING
Net Contents 4 Fld. Ozs.
Manufactured by
COLUMBIA PHARMACY
COR. MAIN & WASHINGTON  SPOKANE WASH

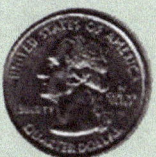

## DR. BONKER'S

*In Scientia est Salutas*

### PEPSIN STOMACH BITTERS

THE BEST KNOWN REMEDY
—FOR—
General Debility,
Biliousness,
Nervousness,
Dyspepsia,
Liver Complaint,
La Grippe,
AND KINDRED DISEASES.

IT ENRICHES THE BLOOD.
IT STRENGTHENS THE NERVES.

Is highly recommended for all diseases requiring certain and efficient tonic, such as Indigestion, Want of Appetite, Loss of Strength, Lack of Energy, Etc.
A mild and safe invigorant for females; a good tonic preparations for ordinary family purposes.

DIRECTIONS.
Wineglassful three times a day before meals. Persons in a delicate condition should begin by taking a small dose and gradually increase, preferably in water.

Dr. Bonker Medicine Co.
CHICAGO, ILL.

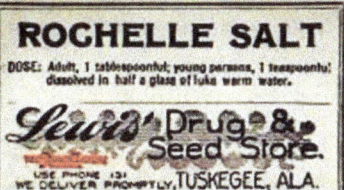

CHAS. A. DREFS, New Drug Store, Deutsche Apotheke,
HOFFMAN'S ANODYNE
280 & 282 Broadway, Cor. Ash St., BUFFALO, N. Y.

### PHILLIPS'
Fragrant Pearlifoam Tooth Wash
None genuine without this signature:
*A. E. Phillips*

MESSING'S PHARMACY.
Deutsche Apotheke,
**POWD. ALUM.**
Pulv. Alum.
78 Broad Street, Stapleton, S. I.

### EYE WATER.
DIRECTIONS.—Put a few drops in the eye occasionally during the day, and especially before retiring at night.
J. B. BROWN, Druggist,
219 North Main St.,    HANNIBAL, MO.

## MRS. H. H. SCRIBNER'S
### RHEUMATIC BALM.

The Best known Remedy for Rheumatism, Colds, Coughs, Sore Throat, Sore Lungs, Sprains, Lameness, Toothache, Etc.

FOR INTERNAL AND EXTERNAL USE.

DIRECTIONS.

DOSE.—Adults, 6 to 8 drops. Children, 2 to 3 drops in one-half cup of hot water well sweetened.
For external use bathe the parts freely, taking a few drops internally at the same time.

PUT UP BY
MRS. H. H. SCRIBNER & SON,
Springfield, Maine.

Price 35 Cents.

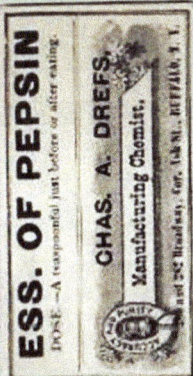

## Act X

# THE CURTAIN CLOSES... & OPENS AGAIN
### Transformation & The Beginnings of a Movement

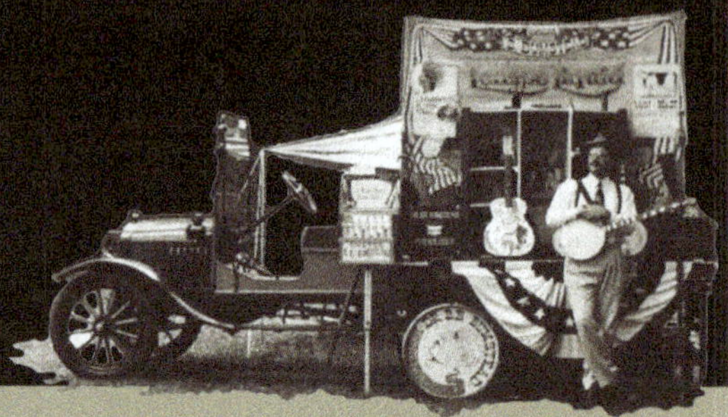

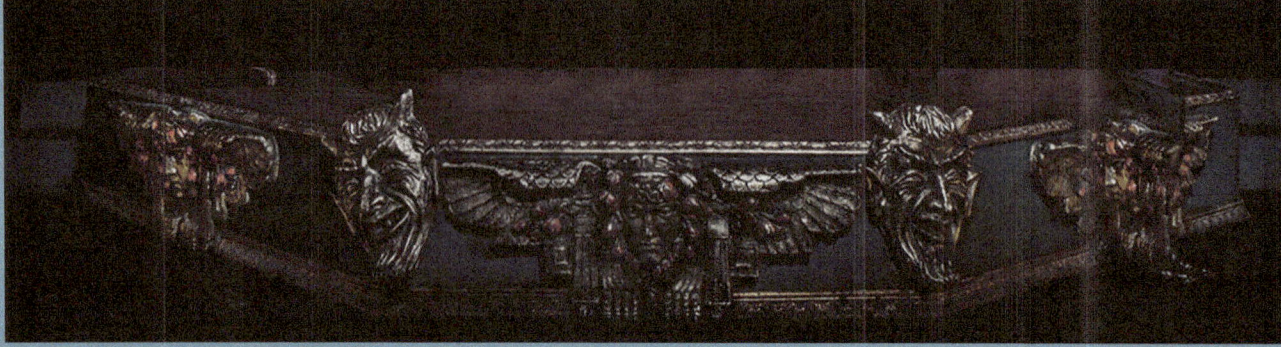

**The Finale**

By the time of the first World War, all but a few of the traveling Medicine Shows had ceased to travel the familiar circuits down the byways and through the out-of-the-way communities of an increasingly urbanized United States. A few shows managed to keep going through the 1920s and 30s, substituting automobiles and trailers for the iconic horses and medicine wagons. Despite all the denigration and unjust legislation, it was not law that spelled their doom, so much as having their plant based remedies co-opted and subsumed by large commercial interests, traveling entertainment of all kinds being replaced by new mediums for entertainment. Their nostrum sales were impacted not just by a shift in the public's opinion of "primitive herbs" versus "modern cures," but also by the rise of giant corporate producers and an increase in the prevalence of mail-order businesses. The very valuable role that Medicine Shows played in bringing entertainment, education and culture to the people of rural American was assumed first by the new medium of radio being fast adopted even in even the most remote settlements, and then in the late 1940s by the introduction of television. One no longer had to walk any further than into their own living rooms to hear and eventually see musicians playing their favorite songs, Native Americans dressed up in tribal costume, lectures of interest, comedians and magicians peddling their jokes and tricks.

This new media was incredibly effective, in part because it adopted so much of the Medicine Show's tried and true formula: the seamless blending of entertainment and a sales message. To this day, "product placement" and "Reality TV" programs fuse and thus confuse dramatic and commercial messages.

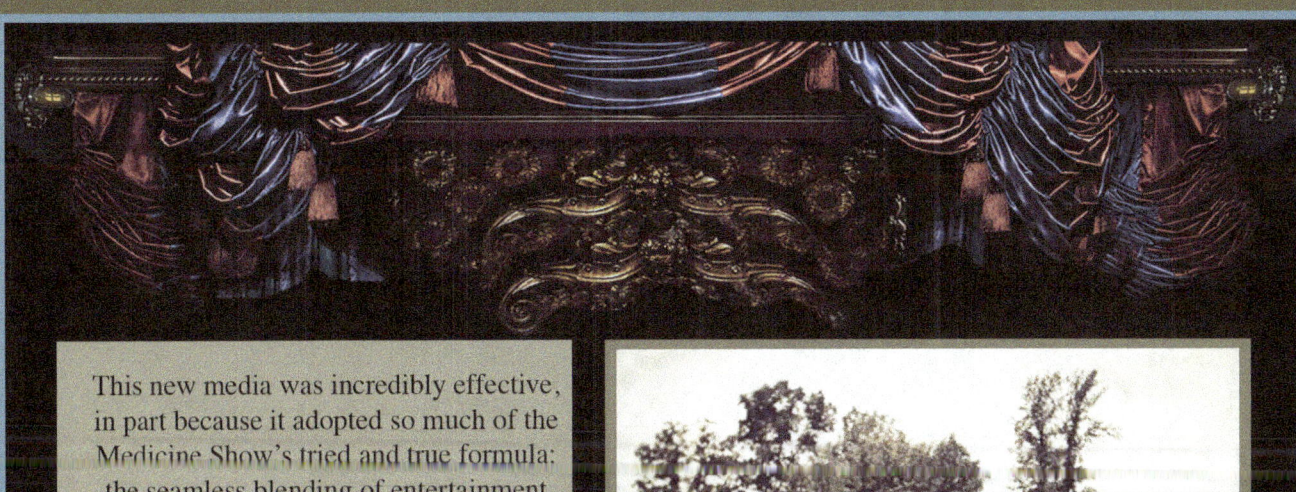
Doc Houck's Medicine Show

Ironically, the mediums that reinforce professional and corporate hegemony – and that trivialize or commercialize natural healing – took their cues from the Medicine Shows that they helped make obsolete: spark people's interest, and use entertainment as a means for getting folks to not only purchase but fundamentally identify with the products offered.

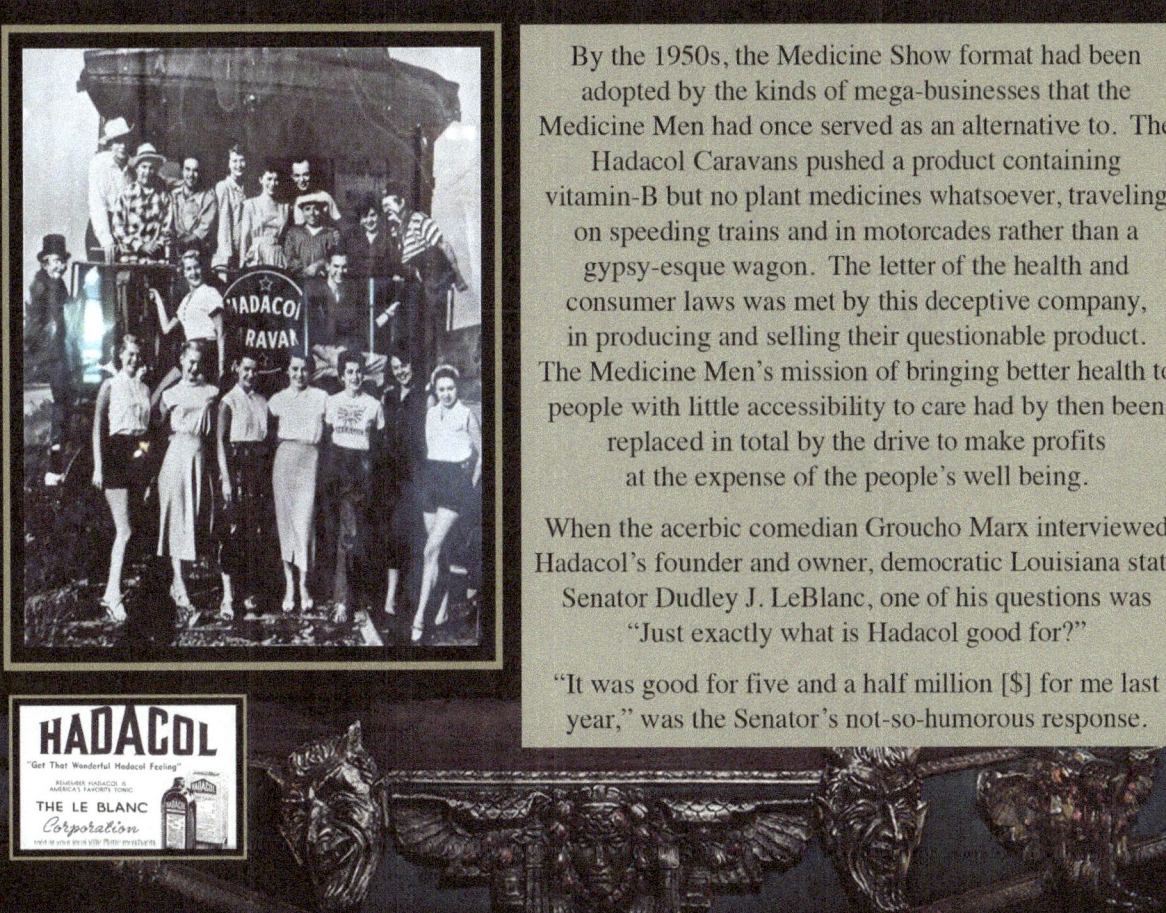

By the 1950s, the Medicine Show format had been adopted by the kinds of mega-businesses that the Medicine Men had once served as an alternative to. The Hadacol Caravans pushed a product containing vitamin-B but no plant medicines whatsoever, traveling on speeding trains and in motorcades rather than a gypsy-esque wagon. The letter of the health and consumer laws was met by this deceptive company, in producing and selling their questionable product. The Medicine Men's mission of bringing better health to people with little accessibility to care had by then been replaced in total by the drive to make profits at the expense of the people's well being.

When the acerbic comedian Groucho Marx interviewed Hadacol's founder and owner, democratic Louisiana state Senator Dudley J. LeBlanc, one of his questions was "Just exactly what is Hadacol good for?"

"It was good for five and a half million [$] for me last year," was the Senator's not-so-humorous response.

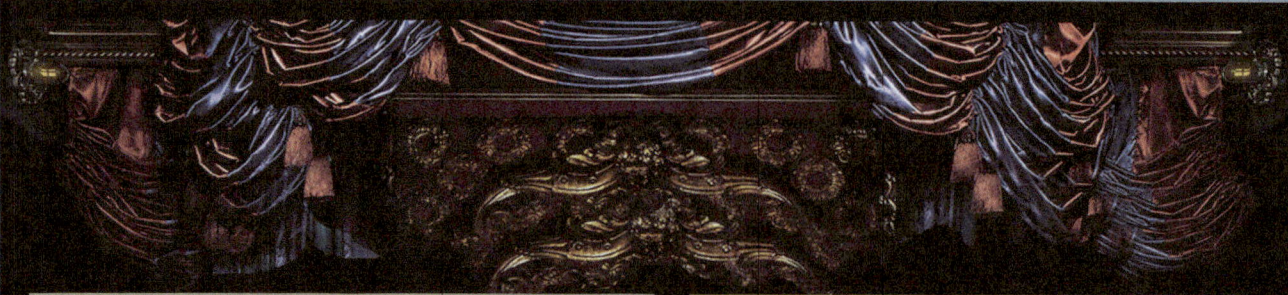

It was only in the 1960s that Medicine Shows were recast in a more positive light, as alternative medicine and holistic health care grew with the development of "alternative lifestyles" and a vibrant "counterculture." After something like 70 years of plant medicines being devalued by a supposedly more sophisticated population, plant medicines were again proving trendy for at a segment of Americans, along with increased interest in healthy foods and tasty cuisine, exercise and yoga, nature/ecology and the environment, bioregionalism, alternative education, spirituality and self-realization. A thriving minority came to relate good livelihood and purpose, good music and good vibes, to good health. Teenagers including myself ran away from the the cities and suburbs, from the relatively uninspired, regimented, black and white reality of the preceding two decades, in a quest to explore alternative communities and natural environs, and similarly choosing to avoid modern mechanistic doctoring in favor of tinctures and teas concocted with highly effective plant parts.

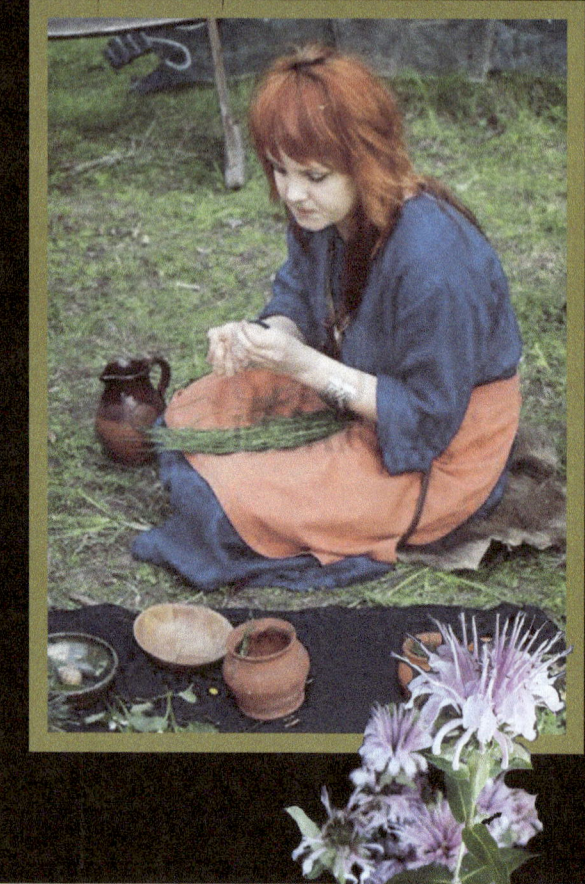

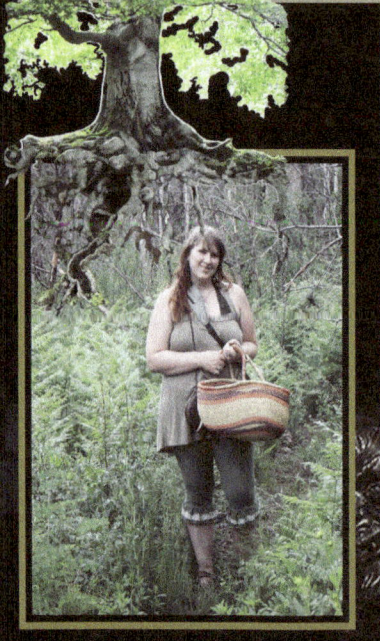

Come the 2010s and beyond, it would still be a combination of governmental legislation and corporate commodification that threatened the ages-long herbal tradition. As proven money-makers, herbs could now be found on the shelves of regular grocery stores, though in many cases industrially processed by companies with few ethics in regards to plant conservation or habitat preservation. Isolated plant compounds have foolishly been promoted over the use of whole plants whose many constituents work together in scarcely understood synergy. Many practicing herbalists began to seek professional registration out of a desire to be accepted as a health care provider in eyes of the larger, conventional society. And yet, thorough it all, something of the old ways – of community service, of conservation, of direct and responsible relationship to the plants, of self empowerment and celebration – not only remained rooted but continued to grow... something of the early "root doctors" and "kitchen witches," "curanderas" and "yerberas," of folk herbalists and those wonderful Traveling Medicine Shows.

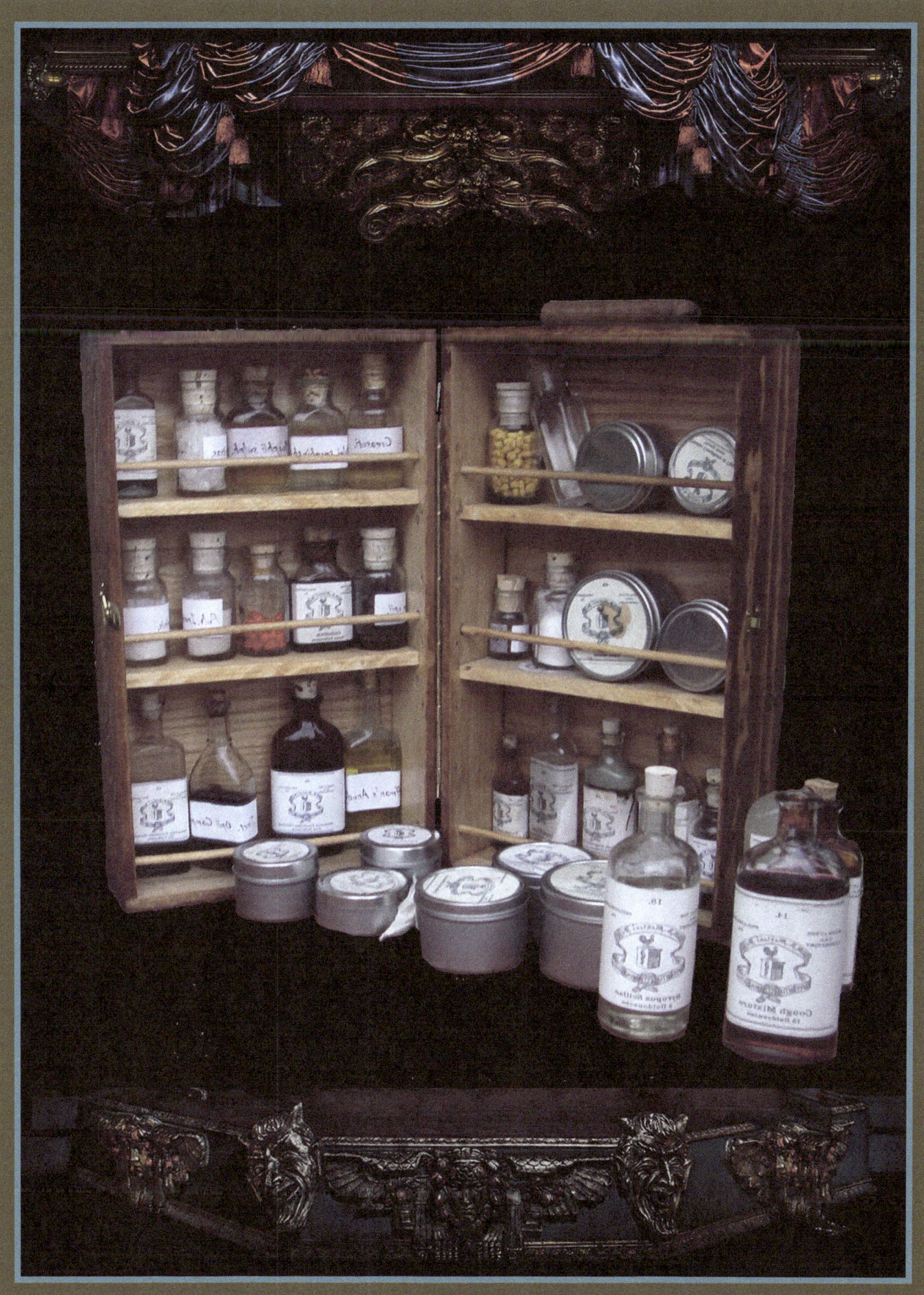

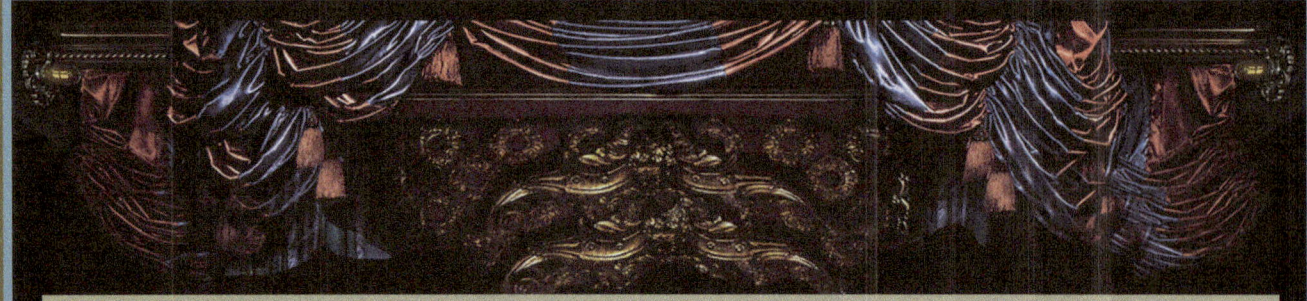

## The Encore

*"Why use chemical drugs when nature in her wisdom and beneficence has provided in her great vegetable laboratories, relief for most of the more common and simple ills of mankind?"*
–Joseph Meyer (1930s)

In most cases, the Medicine Men and Women were working in order to earn a living, yet their primary wish and purpose was to contribute to the quality of people's lives, ease the burdens of their ills and restore them to function and fitness. Few traveling marketers can be dismissed as profiteers, and many were first and foremost devoted to their role as genuine and caring healers.

Throughout its century of optimal prominence, the traveling Medicine Show was the number one threat to the monopoly of licensed health care and pharmaceutical drugs, with the Medicine Man the main counterirritant to the institutionalized prestige and superior status and position of the medical doctor. In the same way, herbs and herbalism today comprise an essential counterbalance to the corporate whitewashing of their often dangerous products, and are attacked precisely because of the challenge them might post to drug sales and profits. The corporate strategy at the time of this writing is to defame or belittle the efficacy of whole plant medicines while marketing products made from isolated or synthesized chemicals and chemical recombinations employing herbal and nature-associated marketing language. Recent legislation continues the attack on herbal preparations made by the owners of small herbal businesses while favoring national and multinational corporate interests.

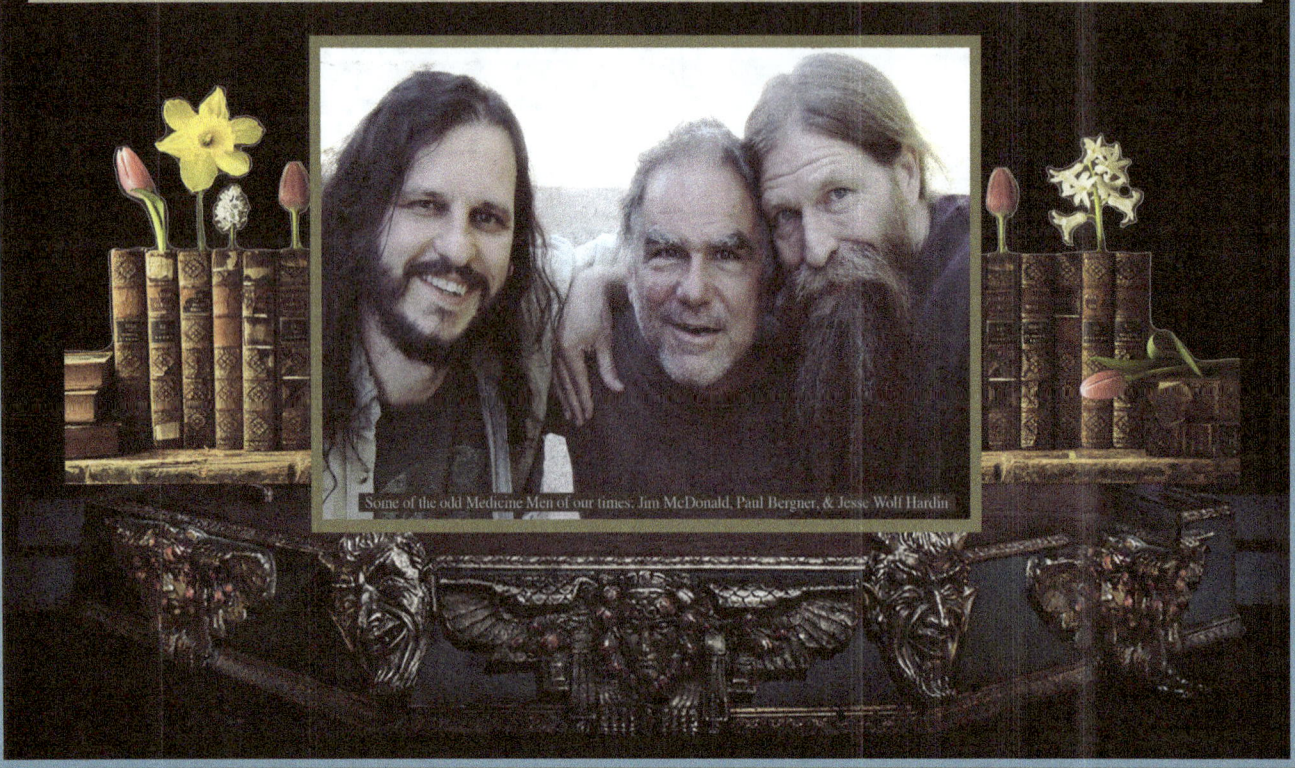

Some of the odd Medicine Men of our times: Jim McDonald, Paul Bergner, & Jesse Wolf Hardin

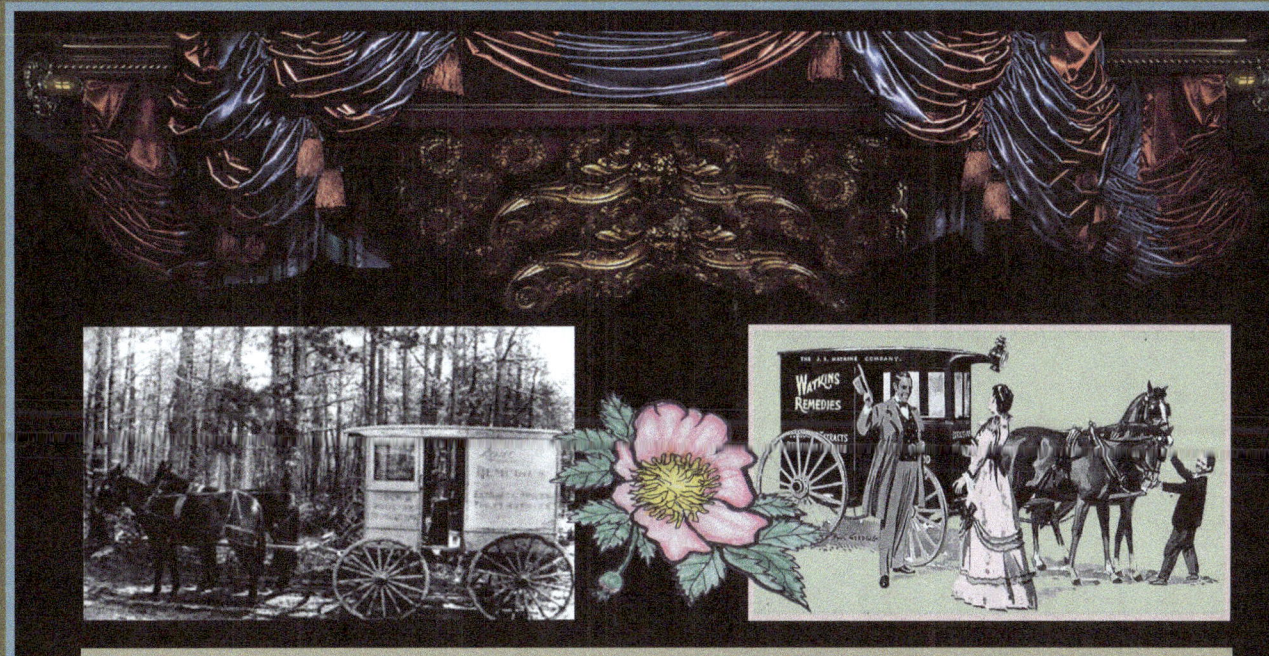

The traveling Medicine Shows, like the practice of herbalism and other forms of natural healing, have served as positive and creative forms of resistance against a life-crushing, de-naturing paradigm. They are, by any definition, truly "alternative." The struggles to keep Medicine Shows and herbalism itself alive have fundamentally been contests over control of our own existence and health, impacting the most intimate relationship of all: that crucial relationship between ourselves and our bodies.

These days, if we do a search for contemporary "Medicine Shows" on the internet we will turn up several pitchmen marketing historic Medicine Show acts as entertainment for conferences, festivals and schools. In most cases these showmen's approach is to reinforce the unfortunate and inaccurate stereotype of the medicine seller as a charming but dishonest bunko artist, fleecing audiences of country rubes with his entertaining tricks and clever lies. More accurately, it is the corporations and their dutiful elected officials who are doing the worst fleecing of the public, while the icon of the Medicine Show represents democratic resistance to dominant cultural dictates, to what are sometimes deleterious synthetic drugs and an institutionalized health care system.

It stands – in truth – as a herald of options, and a call to choice.

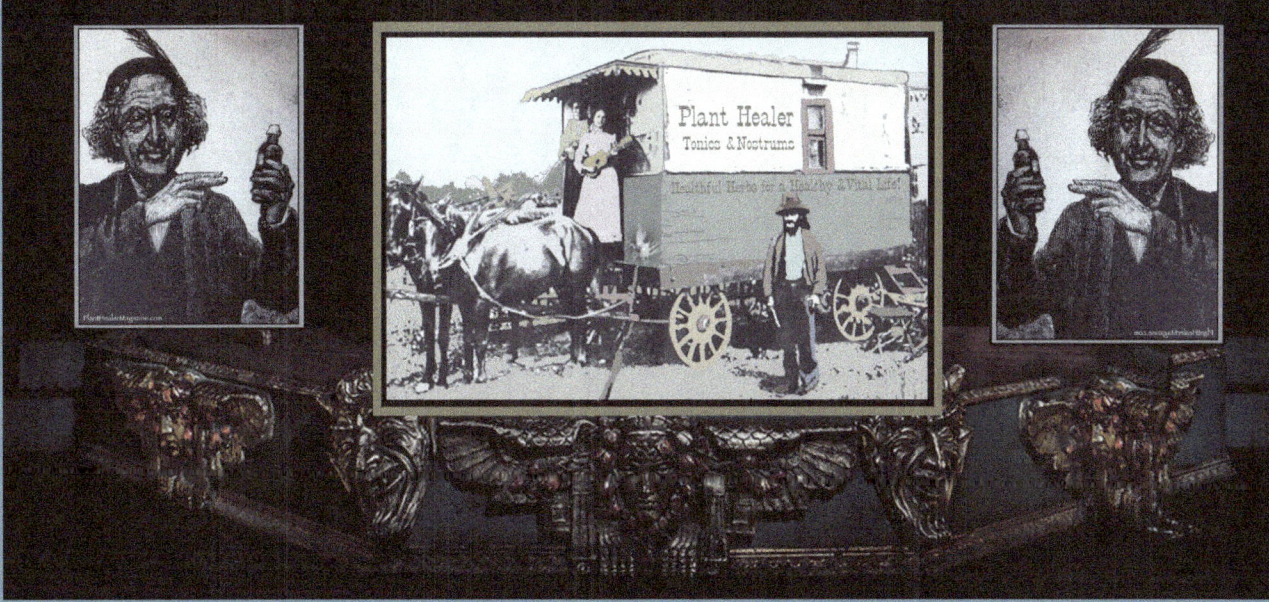

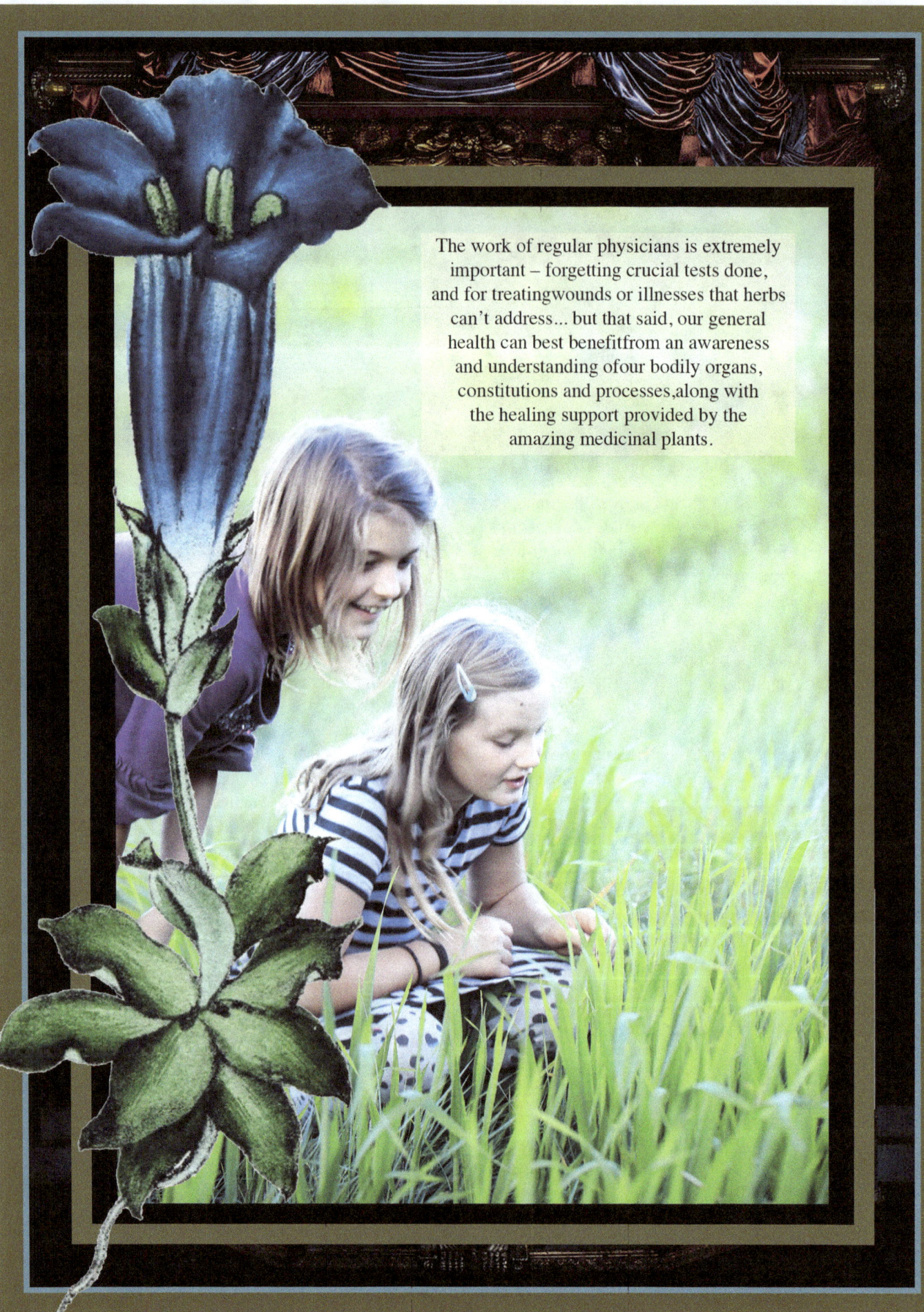

The work of regular physicians is extremely important – forgetting crucial tests done, and for treatingwounds or illnesses that herbs can't address... but that said, our general health can best benefitfrom an awareness and understanding ofour bodily organs, constitutions and processes,along with the healing support provided by the amazing medicinal plants.

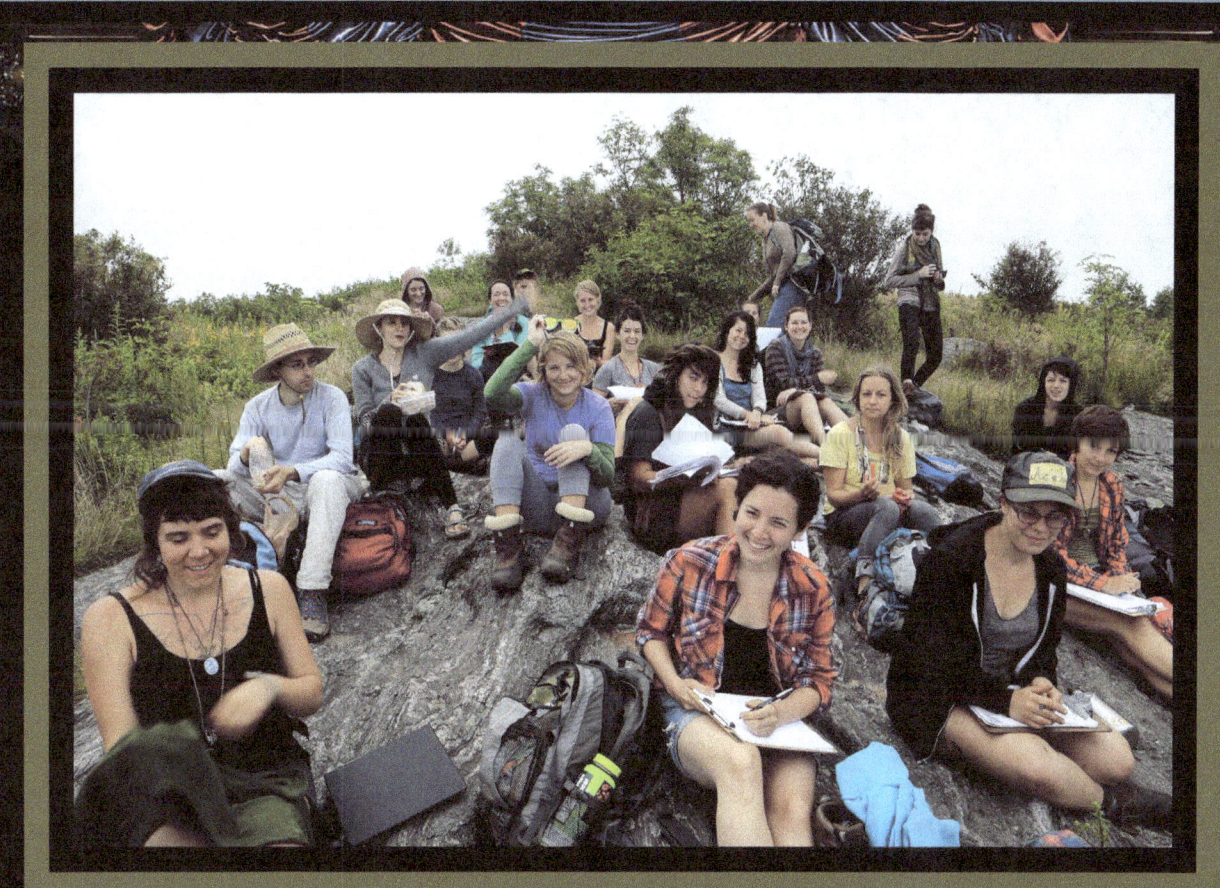

The worst of the Medicine Show products were generally less dangerous than the well accepted drugs being massively prescribed to people in these times. These events for the common folk empowered them to take control of their own health and well being, the opposite of what current advertising seeks to do. We were told by the Medicine Show pitchmen that we had a choice as to how we live our lives, and that we could have an effect on how long and well we survive.

"No man lives forever," the Medicine Man might say, "and in due time age shall have its mortal say. But until that moment it is up to us to make the choices that can extend our stay on this bountiful earth and increase our healthy enjoyment of it." We may or or may not purchase the proffered bottles of "Dr. Goode's," but we take home a feeling of individual empowerment, a bit of curious information and heart-lightening song – a tonic for the spirit that sinks in deep, and lasts long.

The result can be far more than restored respect for the traveling shows of old, or the survival of an archaic tradition of natural healing and community proselytizing. One direct outgrowth is what we have to call a "movement," a reawakening and revitalization that empowers our commitment, change, action, and follow-through. There is a folk herbalism and natural healing renaissance in motion, progressing like a song or dance, creating living alternatives to the what are in the end rather dulling and deadly systems.

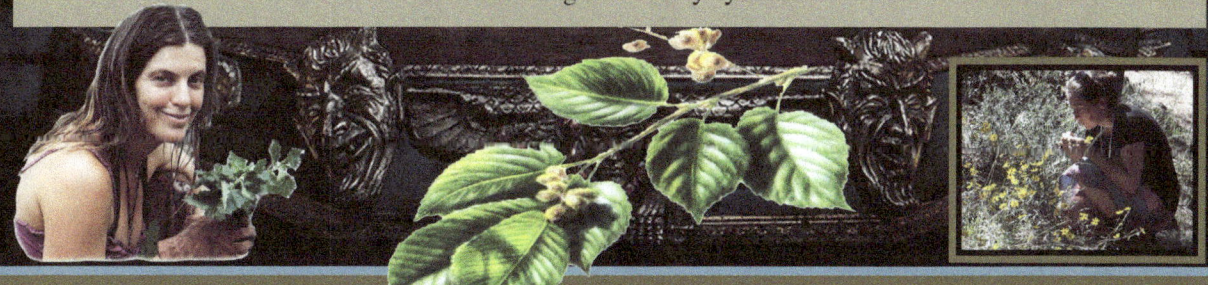

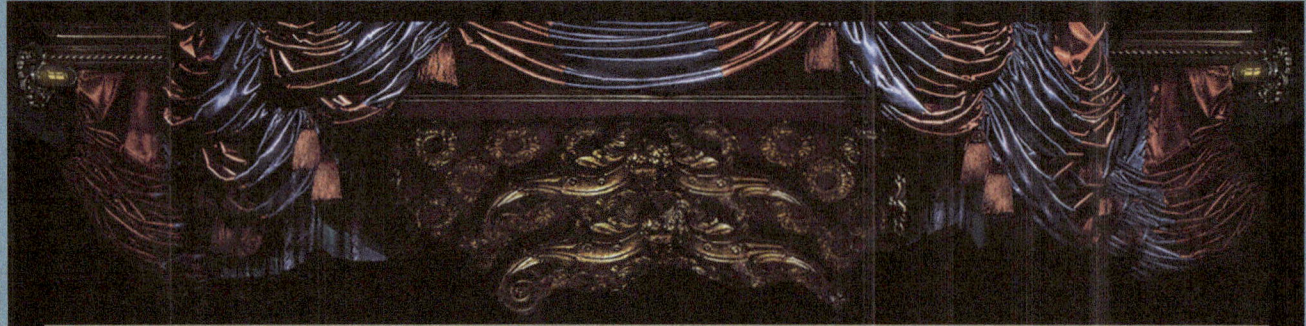

The Medicine Show audience rises as one, and we rise with them! A great howl and clamor erupts from us, the defiantly joyous. We are inspired not just to purchase the natural remedies for our human ailments that we see touted up and down the aisles, but also to seek out the plants from which the medicines are made, to learn those secrets they share, and to use the knowledge gained to help better the health of others. We are inspired not only to affect the healing of our bodies, but also to help heal our kind's emotional beings and troubled psyches, our in many ways unjust society and unhealthy ways of looking at things, the soil and streams, the ecological balance of the natural world from which all does proceed. We sense that we are no longer just an audience, no longer simply witnesses to the rights and wrongs, the ugliness and beauty of our times. As the fervent clapping gets louder, reaching for its sonic climax, we now realize without question that we are also performers and participants, visionaries, artists, activists, helpers and healers charged with the betterment and celebration of life.

*"Hell yeah!,"* someone shouts, snapping the straps on their coveralls, a booted foot excitedly stomping the floor. *"Encore! Encore!"*

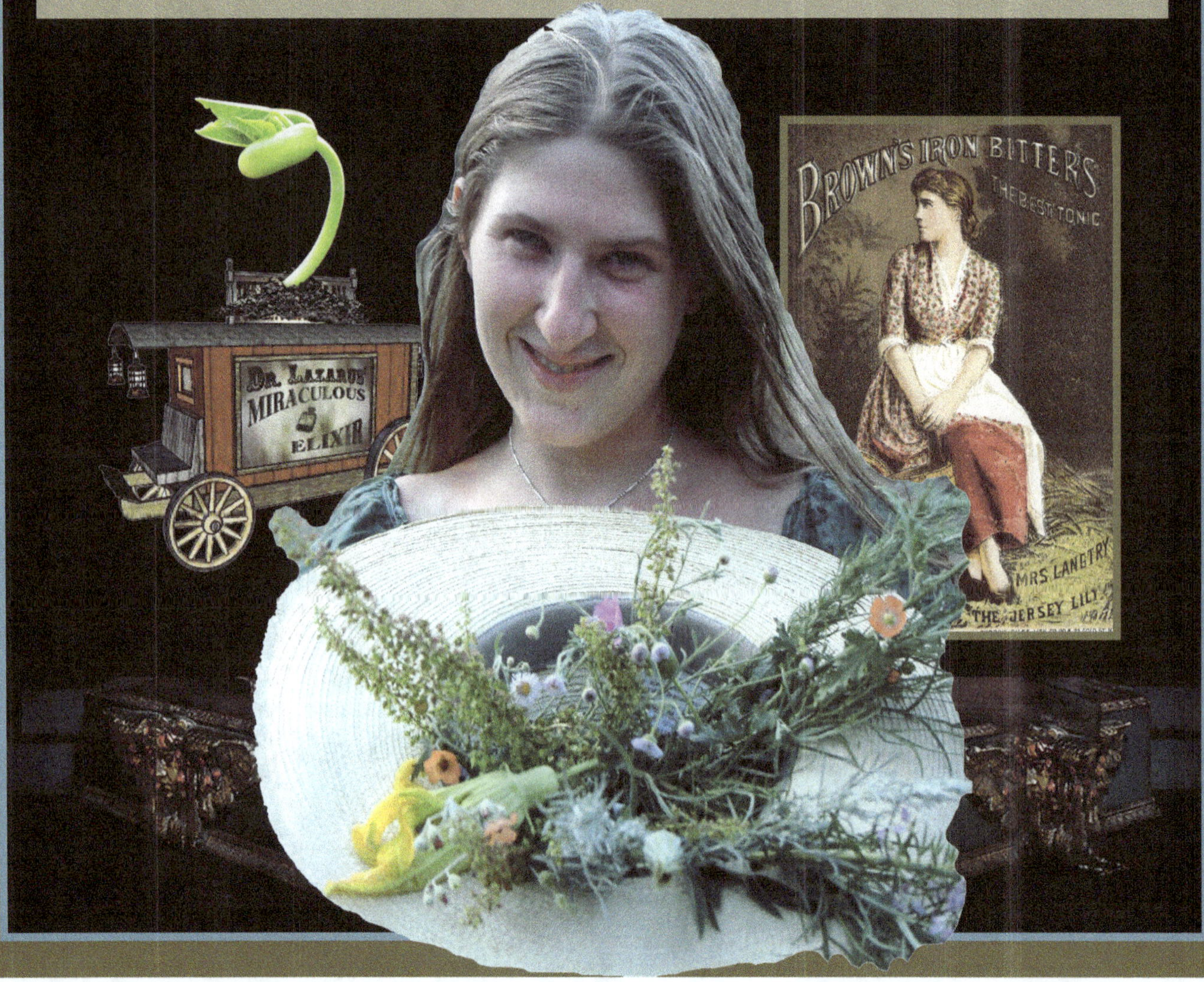

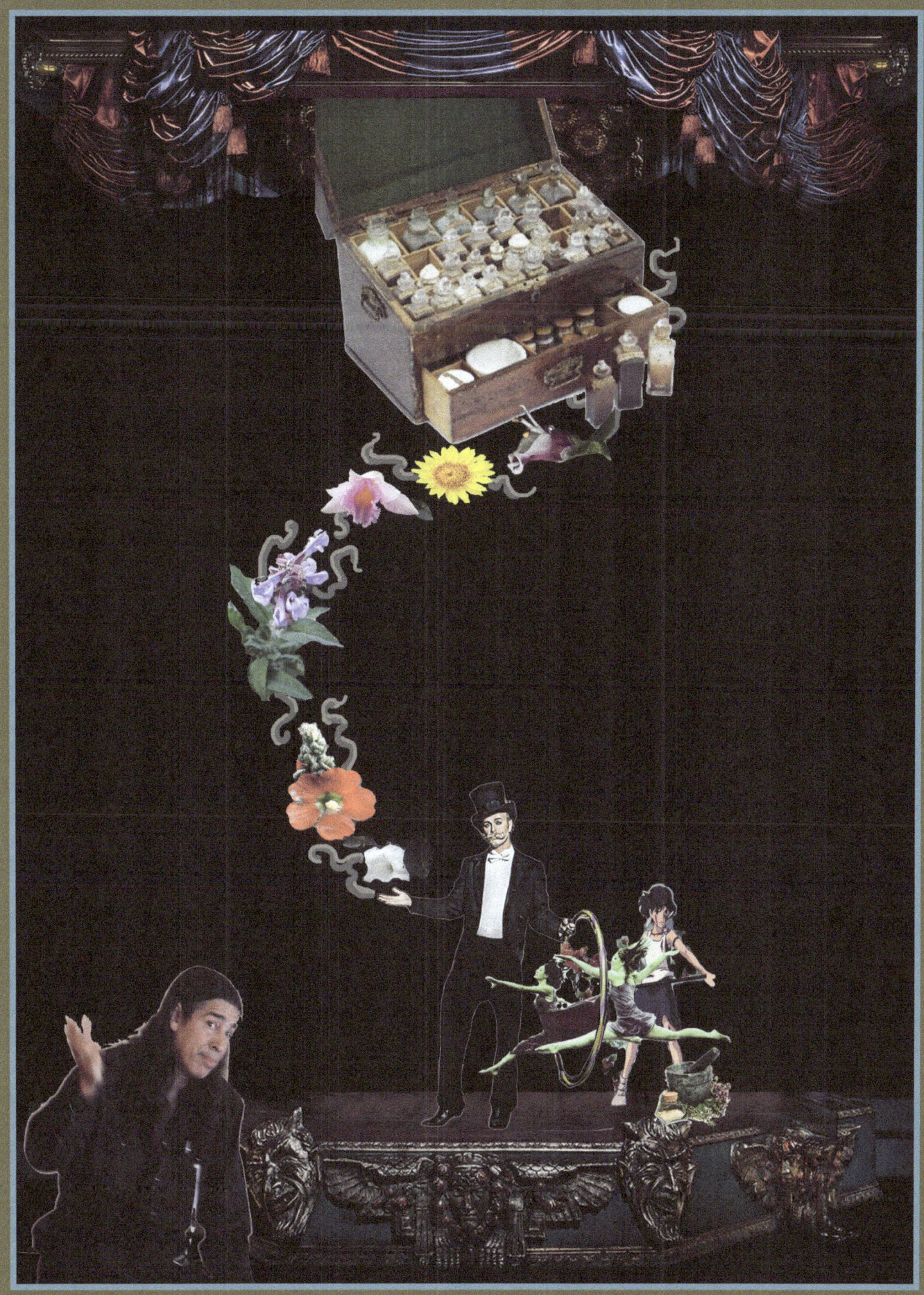

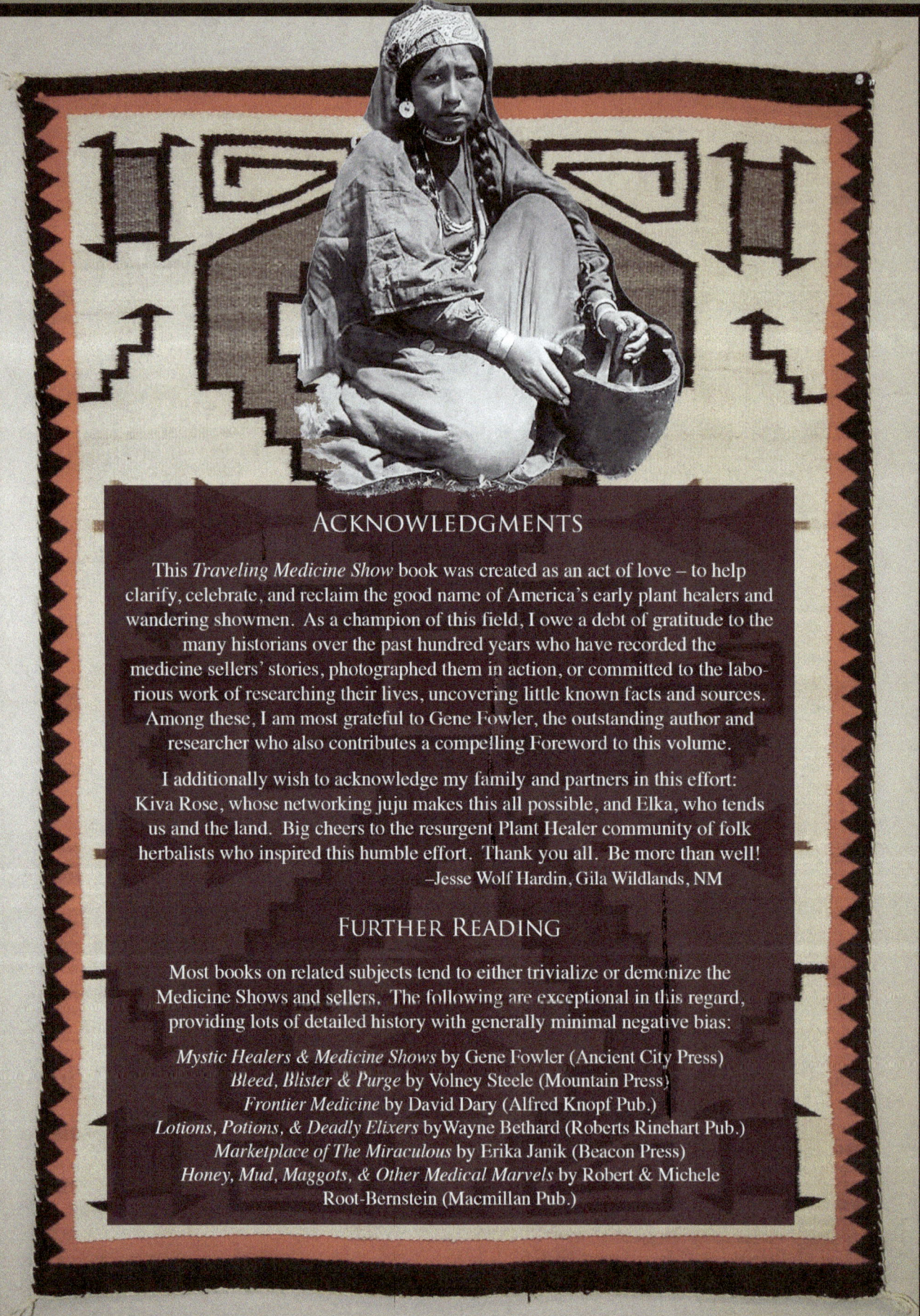

## Acknowledgments

This *Traveling Medicine Show* book was created as an act of love – to help clarify, celebrate, and reclaim the good name of America's early plant healers and wandering showmen. As a champion of this field, I owe a debt of gratitude to the many historians over the past hundred years who have recorded the medicine sellers' stories, photographed them in action, or committed to the laborious work of researching their lives, uncovering little known facts and sources. Among these, I am most grateful to Gene Fowler, the outstanding author and researcher who also contributes a compelling Foreword to this volume.

I additionally wish to acknowledge my family and partners in this effort: Kiva Rose, whose networking juju makes this all possible, and Elka, who tends us and the land. Big cheers to the resurgent Plant Healer community of folk herbalists who inspired this humble effort. Thank you all. Be more than well!
–Jesse Wolf Hardin, Gila Wildlands, NM

## Further Reading

Most books on related subjects tend to either trivialize or demonize the Medicine Shows and sellers. The following are exceptional in this regard, providing lots of detailed history with generally minimal negative bias:

*Mystic Healers & Medicine Shows* by Gene Fowler (Ancient City Press)
*Bleed, Blister & Purge* by Volney Steele (Mountain Press)
*Frontier Medicine* by David Dary (Alfred Knopf Pub.)
*Lotions, Potions, & Deadly Elixers* by Wayne Bethard (Roberts Rinehart Pub.)
*Marketplace of The Miraculous* by Erika Janik (Beacon Press)
*Honey, Mud, Maggots, & Other Medical Marvels* by Robert & Michele Root-Bernstein (Macmillan Pub.)

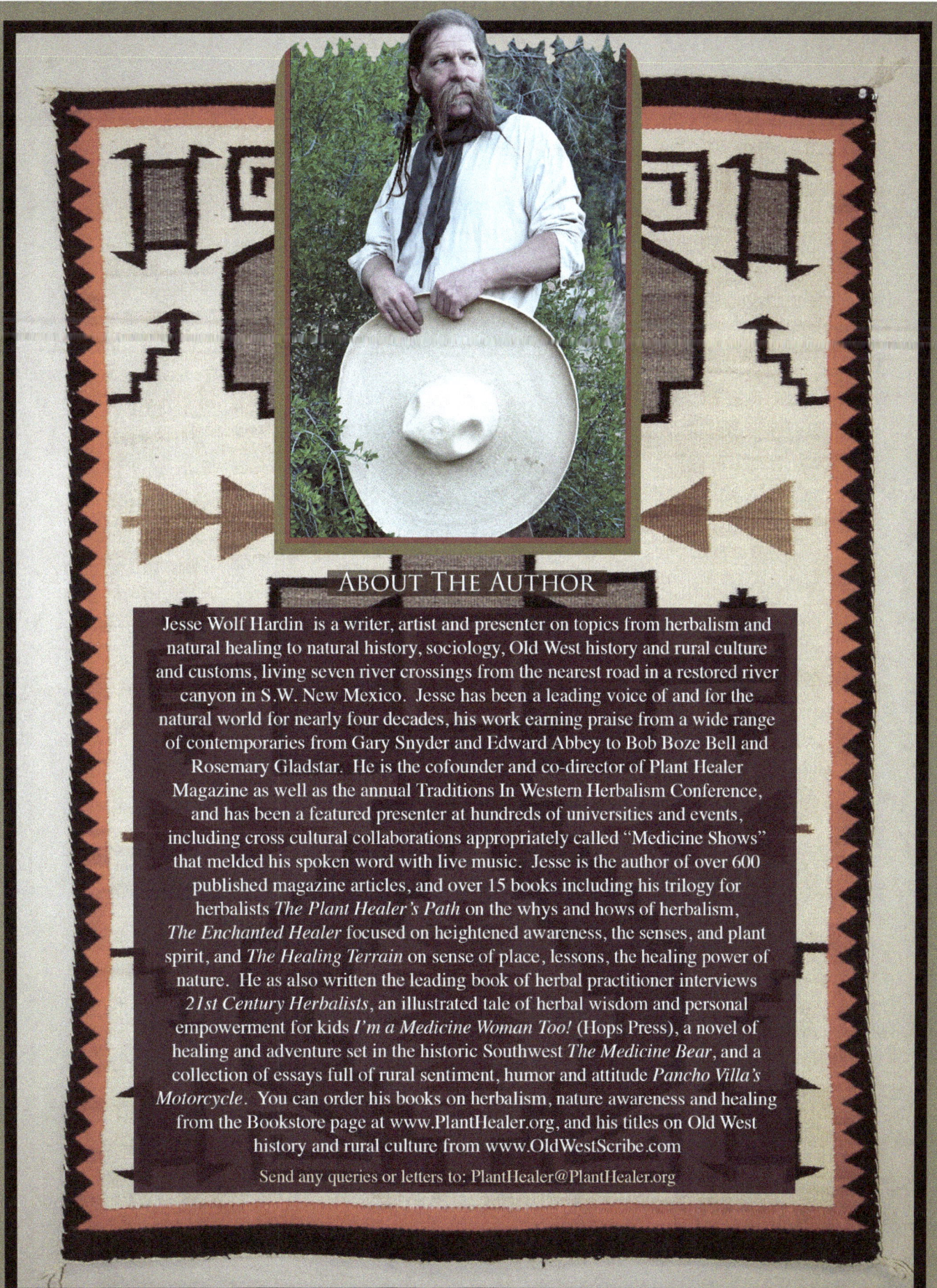

## About The Author

Jesse Wolf Hardin is a writer, artist and presenter on topics from herbalism and natural healing to natural history, sociology, Old West history and rural culture and customs, living seven river crossings from the nearest road in a restored river canyon in S.W. New Mexico. Jesse has been a leading voice of and for the natural world for nearly four decades, his work earning praise from a wide range of contemporaries from Gary Snyder and Edward Abbey to Bob Boze Bell and Rosemary Gladstar. He is the cofounder and co-director of Plant Healer Magazine as well as the annual Traditions In Western Herbalism Conference, and has been a featured presenter at hundreds of universities and events, including cross cultural collaborations appropriately called "Medicine Shows" that melded his spoken word with live music. Jesse is the author of over 600 published magazine articles, and over 15 books including his trilogy for herbalists *The Plant Healer's Path* on the whys and hows of herbalism, *The Enchanted Healer* focused on heightened awareness, the senses, and plant spirit, and *The Healing Terrain* on sense of place, lessons, the healing power of nature. He as also written the leading book of herbal practitioner interviews *21st Century Herbalists*, an illustrated tale of herbal wisdom and personal empowerment for kids *I'm a Medicine Woman Too!* (Hops Press), a novel of healing and adventure set in the historic Southwest *The Medicine Bear*, and a collection of essays full of rural sentiment, humor and attitude *Pancho Villa's Motorcycle*. You can order his books on herbalism, nature awareness and healing from the Bookstore page at www.PlantHealer.org, and his titles on Old West history and rural culture from www.OldWestScribe.com

Send any queries or letters to: PlantHealer@PlantHealer.org

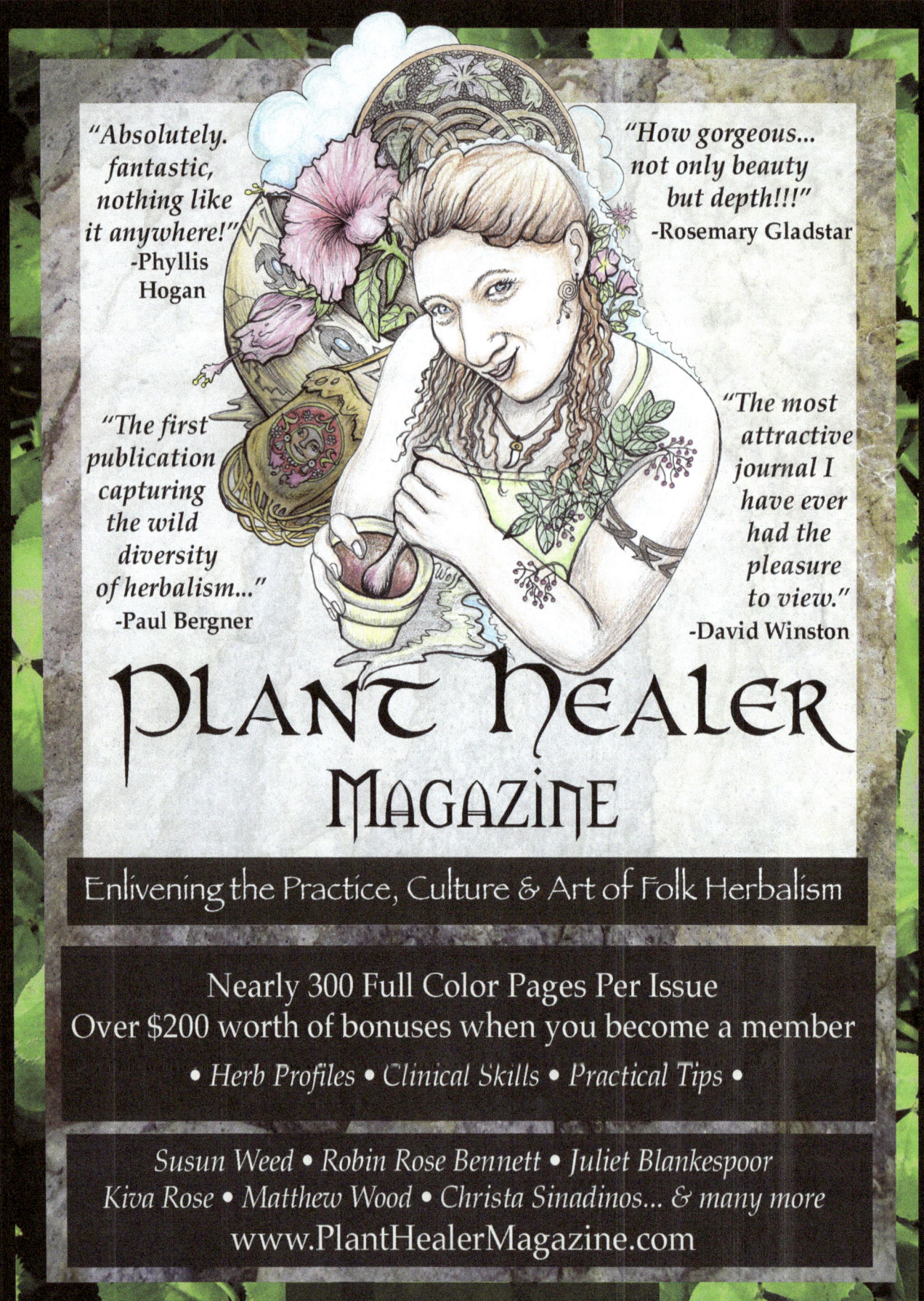

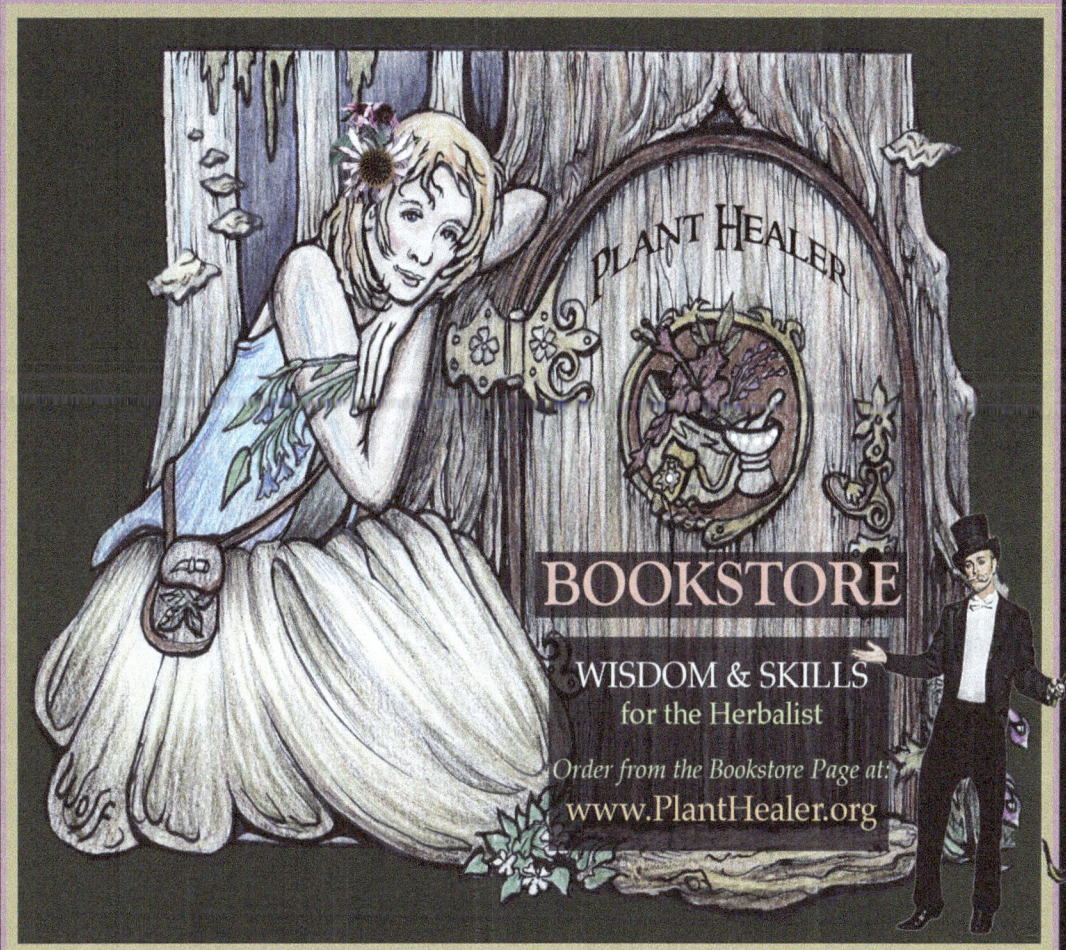

# PLANT HEALER
## BOOKSTORE
### WISDOM & SKILLS
for the Herbalist

*Order from the Bookstore Page at:*
www.PlantHealer.org

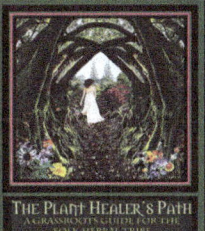
The Plant Healer's Path
Softcover 304p. $29

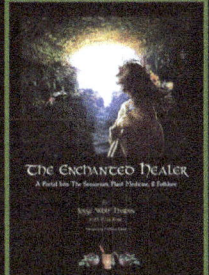
The Enchanted Healer
All Color 295p. $39

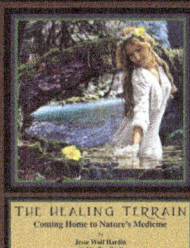
The Healing Terrain
Softbound 307p. $29

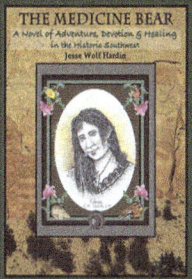
Fiction for Herbalists
Softbound 375p. $18

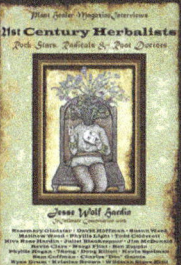
Interviews w/Herbalists
Softbound 376p. $39

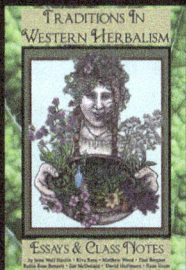
Traditions in Western
Herbalism
Softbound 380p. $29

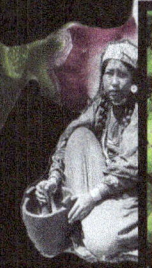 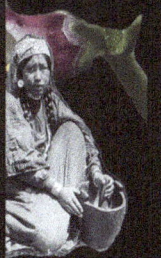
Herbal Wisdom Treasury
Plant Healer 2010-14
Softbound 340p. $29

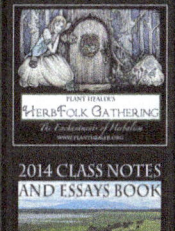
Essays & Class Notes
Ebooks
$19

# A Long & Treasured Tradition

# Of Bringing You Good Medicine